PREVENTION DIARIES

PREVENTION DIARIES

The Practice and Pursuit of Health for All

Larry Cohen

OXFORD
UNIVERSITY PRESS

OXFORD
UNIVERSITY PRESS

Oxford University Press is a department of the University of Oxford. It furthers
the University's objective of excellence in research, scholarship, and education
by publishing worldwide. Oxford is a registered trade mark of Oxford University
Press in the UK and certain other countries.

Published in the United States of America by Oxford University Press
198 Madison Avenue, New York, NY 10016, United States of America.

© Oxford University Press 2017

Library of Congress Cataloging-in-Publication Data
Names: Cohen, Larry, 1947 May 21– author.
Title: Prevention diaries : the practice and pursuit of health for all / Larry Cohen.
Description: Oxford ; New York : Oxford University Press, 2017. |
Includes bibliographical references and index.
Identifiers: LCCN 2016019046 (print) | LCCN 2016030918 (ebook) |
ISBN 9780190623821 (hardback : acid-free paper) | ISBN 9780190623838 (e-book) |
ISBN 9780190623845 (e-book)
Subjects: LCSH: Medicine, Preventive—United States. | Public health—United States. |
Medical policy—United States. | Medical care—Safety measures—United States. |
BISAC: MEDICAL / Public Health.
Classification: LCC RA445 .C54 2016 (print) | LCC RA445 (ebook) |
DDC 362.10973—dc23
LC record available at https://lccn.loc.gov/2016019046

3 5 7 9 8 6 4 2
Printed by Sheridan Books, Inc., United States of America

CONTENTS

INTERLUDE
CANCER

INTERLUDE
CONEY ISLAND

SPECIAL THANK YOU

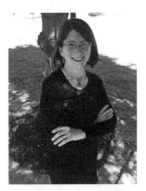

Throughout the six years of intense creation of this book, Anne Giunta Paniagua served as co-writer, editor, and curator of my ideas, invaluably helping to shape my vision into *Prevention Diaries*. Anne is a freelance writer, editor, and translator who lives in San Francisco and southern France with her husband and two daughters. My profound thanks go to Anne for her commitment to purpose, attention to detail, passion for prevention, commitment to social justice, deep reflection, and constant patience.

NOTE OF APPRECIATION

The *Prevention Diaries* draws on my learning, experiences, and work from the beginning of my career through the creation and nearly two decades of the Prevention Institute. I am extraordinarily grateful to my colleagues and co-workers for the breadth of their support in our shared work and in the development of this book. I'm also grateful to the numerous advocates and collaborators, whose passion and vision advance health, prevention, and equity, and to make it possible to believe in a future where *everyone* is healthy and safe.

My gratitude goes to the entire Prevention Institute staff who many times needed to do more because I was writing this book, and to our Board of Directors who saw the value of this endeavor. I am particularly grateful to those who gave ongoing support in the creation of *Prevention Diaries*, providing insight, editing, writing, research, guidance, administrative support and organization: Anna Realini, Sana Chehimi, Michi Arguedas, Jessica Berthold, Juliet Sims, Leslie Mikkelsen, Rachel Davis, Manal Aboelata, Ilan Friedmann-Grunstein, Perla Camacho, Meb Byrne, and Raquel Toledo.

Numerous colleagues and Prevention Institute staff contributed by reviewing and editing chapters and providing knowledge, data, and vision: Annie Lyles, Caroline Guzman, Daphne Miller, Janani Srikantharajah, Janet Pan, Julie Leung, Kinnari Shah, Larissa Estes, Lily Swartz, Linda

Nkemere, Mariel Harding, Maureen Silva, Nicole Schneider, Nikta Akhavan, Rachel Bennett, Rea Panares, Rebekah Kharrazi, Sandra Viera, Sarah Mittermaier, Sharon Murriquez, Sheila Savannah, Veonna Washington, Victoria Nichols, Will Haar, Xavier Morales, Xenia Shih.

Barb Alberson, Carol Runyon, Dick Jackson, Dinesh Mohan, Jean Nudelman, Judy Derman, Kate Pastor, Kelly Brownell, Linda Degutis, Lori Dorfman, Mari Egan, Marion Nestle, Mark Fenton, Mark Pertschuk, Mike Pastor, Peggy Mohan, Shelli Stidham, Steve Wirtz.

And a special thank you to Chad Zimmerman, my editor at Oxford University Press, for his tireless skill, commitment, and flexibility.

IN SUPPORT OF

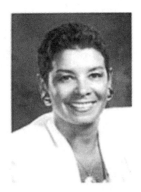

Royalties from *Prevention Diaries* will be used for the Prevention Institute's *Dr. Beverly Coleman Miller Fellowship* supporting post-graduate and graduate students, particularly those of color, to continue Beverly's mission of health equity through youth violence prevention, mental health, health system transformation, and social justice. Beverly was a youth violence prevention pioneer, a friend, a colleague, and an inspiration. She emphasized that every breath matters, and in our limited breaths, every one of us can have a profound impact in improving the world.

[1]

PRELUDE TO PREVENTION

PEOPLE "GET" PREVENTION

Taking care of my two-year-old nephew, Milo, for the weekend, I quickly go through the house, hiding the dishwashing detergent and other chemical cleaners and inserting guards into the sockets so he doesn't get hurt. On the first day, I have to say "no" a lot, as I discover things that shouldn't be within his reach. He drops toys down heater vents and climbs into the fireplace. Pretty soon, most of the house is childproofed, and he's busy playing with the new delights he finds around him—the cooking utensils I deliberately left available for him to discover—and he soon goes out to the fenced-in section of the yard, digging in the sand, filling a bottle of water through a funnel, and smelling the lavender. I notice that with mostly innocuous surroundings, it's much easier for him to stay safe, and I hardly have to say "no" to him at all. He's much happier this way, and so am I.

It's a natural instinct to look out for the health and well-being of family and friends. And, as we are reminded whenever they are befallen with illness or injury, few things matter more. As humans, we have a natural understanding that people flourish in a safer, healthier environment, and when it comes to people we love, we're naturally inclined to put them in situations that minimize their risks. In this way, we get prevention. Just as I tried to protect Milo from harm, we all want living conditions that foster health and safety, particularly for those close to us.

On a personal level, we understand that by eating and sleeping well, staying active, reducing stress, and getting medical care, when necessary, we'll live longer, healthier lives. That's what makes it so stunning that, as a country and society, we often encourage the opposite of what our own

1

instincts tell us to do. Consequently, people have to work harder than ever to avoid being among the growing numbers plagued by chronic diseases, injuries, and premature death. Why is this? Do we *all* lack discipline and self-control? Behavior is a factor, but it goes beyond that.

Our best intentions and efforts often clash with the experiences we have in our communities, the products that are available, and the actions of businesses and mainstream media—all of which greatly determine our opportunities for health and safety. When we walk out our doors, are we greeted by an abundance of healthy, affordable, and culturally desirable food or a proliferation of fast-food chains? Are there safe parks with children playing and elders walking? Do we see rolling landscapes or are we confronted with billboards, glamorizing alcohol and tobacco's false promises of sexual prowess, power, and vitality? Do televisions and radios blare with pharmaceutical ads promising an instant cure (just beware of the side effects—"nausea, impotence, and in serious cases may include death")?

The answers to these questions lie at the heart of our ability to actually lead healthy, safe lives. Most of these challenges are more difficult in communities that have experienced discrimination and disinvestment, where residents almost always bear the greatest burden of illness and injury—not because they lack the moral fiber, discipline, or common sense to make good decisions but rather because they systematically lack access to resources and opportunities for health, and it's not by accident.

IN THE FIRST PLACE

No one grows up hoping to be a prevention director. In the 1980s, while working in a county health department in northern California, I was offered a chance to pioneer a new approach: to grapple with multiple health and safety issues simultaneously in the role of director of prevention. I asked myself what prevention was all about and what I could accomplish. After all, I had set out to work in government because I wanted to have a decisive impact, and I cared deeply about fairness and justice, promoting the kinds of changes that particularly benefited those who most greatly needed increased opportunities and support. Yet my impression was that prevention was mushy. I feared it would translate to inconsequential work, like putting up highway billboards saying, "Drink milk." I accepted the position but needed to discover—or create—an approach through which I could have a deeper impact.

Shortly after I started my new job, a prominent local entrepreneur suffered a major heart attack. Ordinarily, he would have gone to a fancy private hospital, but he had his heart attack right across the street from the public hospital. Although the initial prognosis was poor, the excellent care resulted in a quick and near-complete recovery. This led to the county board of supervisors extolling the virtues of their healthcare facilities and the quality treatment they dispensed. As their meeting was winding down, one elected official, who had a background as a school health educator, asked the director of health, "But what about prevention? Do we do anything for preventing heart attacks?"

This was a great question. The entrepreneur had garnered local fame for both his extraordinary business savvy and his demonstrated lack of prudence in taking care of himself; his personal motto was, "Rich food, big cigars, why walk?" And he was known for his intensely busy and stressful lifestyle. But the expectation of men was to be invincible.

I was anxious to hear what my new boss, the director of health, would say. Perhaps it could help shape my understanding of prevention and of my job. Without missing a beat, the health director responded, "Prevention? Yes, of course. We've got brochures." Holding up a stack of flyers titled, Staying Fit and Heart Healthy, he exclaimed, "We have these!"

"Brochures?" I thought, "That's inadequate. People need more than a piece of paper to change their habits." When health officials focused on treatment, they thought about quality. But prevention was an afterthought, and no one focused on its quality or effectiveness.

BEYOND BROCHURES

Suddenly it became clear to me that I could have a much more significant impact by helping people prevent illnesses and injuries *in the first place*—before they happened. The US healthcare system, along with most people's ways of thinking, has been oriented around fixing illnesses and injuries *after* they occur. Clinical professionals are well trained to treat illnesses and injuries, and having access to their treatment and resources is necessary and, in many cases, life-saving. But this system is expensive and does nothing to reduce the occurrence and burden of the top-five killers in the United States—heart disease, cancer, stroke, respiratory diseases, and injuries—or the proliferation of diabetes. There are also the burdens of family suffering, reduced business productivity, overwhelmed clinical systems, and strained public resources.

In fact, our healthcare system costs a *lot*. One out of $6 of the US gross domestic product is spent on healthcare, and that number is continually going up.[1] Of even greater concern, trends show that even with this spending, children are likely to live shorter lives than their parents.[2] With a mounting evidence base making the case for prevention, and with 75 percent of healthcare money devoted to treating potentially preventable conditions, the United States nevertheless continues to spend over 96 cents of every healthcare dollar treating illnesses and injuries *after* they occur,[3] with fewer than 4 cents of every dollar invested in preventing them.[4]

Increasingly I also understood that, as a nation, we could save lives and protect people from unnecessary anguish by creating and promoting a complementary approach to after-the-fact treatment, one emphasizing high-quality prevention strategies aimed at a community level. Now, decades later, I know firsthand that by taking earlier action, we *can* prevent many people's health and safety challenges, including heart attacks, injuries, and many types of cancer, and that's especially important for the most disadvantaged. The efforts I've been involved in have also confirmed that prevention offers a much smarter fiscal model. California's tobacco-control program, for example, saved $134 billion in personal healthcare costs from 1989 to 2008, while spending only $2.4 billion on the program—a 5,500 percent return on investment.[5]

PERVERSE INCENTIVES

My first prevention office was a converted broom closet, complete with utility sink. As our department's interventions became successful and our staff grew, we moved—this time to a converted underground parking garage. Such accommodations suited me fine, but they also revealed the weak commitment the health leaders had toward developing a strong prevention approach. Even as my work progressed, I wondered: Why had they hired me for this job? I had no specific prevention background; surely there were better candidates available.

In fact, I was recruited because the county was conducting an experiment in partnership with the federal government. Its healthcare agency had a hospital and clinical services division, which sat alongside a separate public health division. The clinical services division almost entirely served patients with federally paid insurance (Medicaid) and was transforming to a "capitation system," in which payment for treating these patients would be a set amount agreed to at the beginning of each year for the entire patient population. (Historically healthcare providers in the United States have been paid in an itemized fashion by specific clinical service delivered.) In order to receive payment under Medicaid, healthcare providers had to submit voluminous reimbursement forms for each patient's diagnosis and treatment.

Instead, the county agency I worked for was betting they could win by agreeing to an experiment of lump-sum annual payments from the government, eliminating the need for detailed financial reports. The clinical providers could operate more efficiently and do what they were meant to do, focus on care, not on pushing papers. The federal government would pay less—only 90 percent of the past year's total amount.

This was the first time such a system was attempted in the United Sates. The incentives for this deal had nothing at all to do with prevention. One imaginative county physician recognized that if they received the same amount of money regardless of what they were doing, and regardless of whether people got sick, there would no longer be the typical *perverse incentive*—a system in which funding increased as the rate and severity of illness and injury rose. In fact, for an agency whose responsibilities included promoting health, this represented an opportunity to align its prevention goals with its financial strategy. Though this made sense, county officials weren't convinced the changes would have significant impact. So rather than go through a hiring process or conduct a formal search, the department just filled the position (with me) through a transfer from a different department. I got my job most unceremoniously.

The major benefit of the switch from fee-for-service to capitation was an open door to prevention strategies, which substantially reduced misery, loss of life, and financial costs. A lot of my early work revolved around identifying and promoting effective prevention strategies. For example, a local young boy living in a smog-filled industrial area suffered frequent asthma attacks. The emergency department providers who repeatedly treated him pointed out that it would be cheaper, more effective, and more humane to buy him an air purifier.

Under the old system, the county couldn't submit claims for such items; it could only be reimbursed for emergency care. For me, this typified another of our healthcare system's perverse incentives—the system encouraged short-term profitability as opposed to health and long-term sustainability. I could see that we needed to systematically realign our priorities, incentives, and payment structures so they synchronized with wellness, not ever-more complex, costly treatments. This would also reduce workloads for clinical providers, improve care for those who really needed it, and help healthcare institutions maintain financial viability, while contributing more resources to community prevention strategies that encourage health and safety. In this case, the capitation system allowed providers to invest more wisely. The health department bought him an air purifier, which improved his immediate environment, helped control his asthma, and saved the county considerable money. (Of course, there's far more to do about asthma, both at the individual level and community efforts, but this was at least a first move in a new direction.)

Historically in the United States, prevention hasn't been prioritized, and, furthermore, virtually no attention has been paid to fostering a systematic, quality prevention approach. For decades, the national prevention model relied primarily on educating people about health and safety risks, hoping they would magically change their behavior. As well intended as educational efforts are, they can never be very effective without simultaneously changing home and community environments, social norms, policies, and institutions. Establishing a broader view—"beyond brochures," we might say—is critical. Research has shown it is unrealistic to expect that simply warning people about a danger will be sufficient to help them change their long-standing habits or avoid unhealthy exposures on their own.[6] A quality prevention approach is one in which education is part of a well-designed, sustained, comprehensive effort to broadly improve community environments, social norms, institutional practices, and policies.

Recognizing this, I went to work identifying clues that pointed to underlying conditions in the community environment that influence what people are exposed to and how they behave, for better or worse.[7] My premise was that, by altering these conditions, we could help create an environment that would truly support everyone in their quest to be healthy and safe. Large institutions like corporations and government would need to play a role, since they influence what's available, accessible, and attractive in our culture and communities. Expanding beneficial options and policies in all community environments would provide everyone a foundation that supports health—fostering a new norm.

Based on these clues, my department launched a number of broad prevention initiatives at the county level, including the following.

- We created the nation's first consistent multicity no-smoking laws, which helped usher in nationwide smoking bans that made *not smoking* the norm.
- Our staff partnered with local hospitals and governments to help make car seat usage standard practice, as we had all seen too many infants and young children rushed by ambulance to hospitals, injured in crashes due to not using car seats.
- We instituted support for families and youth, including encouragement for community strategies to prevent suicide. Emphasizing the links among work, worth, and health, at a time of corporate downsizing, we partnered with unemployment offices to engage out-of-work people as volunteers in peer support efforts. The volunteer's role was to help peers survive the painful, risky period until they, hopefully, worked again, linking them with needed services, including counseling, suicide prevention, and health services. The initiative was at least as constructive for the volunteers as it was for their peers, helping them feel useful and involved.

Because our team worked on so many different topics, we were able—perhaps for the first time in the United States—to take the knowledge from one prevention issue and apply it to others.

These relatively quick achievements affirmed that preventing problems on a wide scale can have a much greater health impact than after-the-
fact treatment can. Decades later, even small, yet incremental measures
like providing an air purifier still aren't commonplace. Effective strategies
to reduce air pollution at the source haven't been widely implemented. The
good news, though, is that the case for prevention is timeless and never
expires: it is really a matter of taking the simple, intuitive lessons from
daily life and applying them to all systems, including public health, clinical care, business, and government. As with asthma, for example, much of
what it takes to sustain health and safety goes beyond clinical care.

Such successes also confirmed my conviction that making positive
changes to the *environments* where people live, work, and play with their families expands the opportunity and likelihood of health. This relates to practices
such as promoting mass transit, walking, and bicycling; making affordable,
nutritious, and culturally appropriate food easily accessible; rethinking how
communities are physically designed; getting people reconnected to each
other; lowering rates of violence; creating living wage jobs; and developing
quality education. By providing the same healthful opportunities for *everyone*, communities can protect the well-being of all their members.

AND NOW, *PREVENTION DIARIES*

Encouraged by the successes I had seen at the county level, I launched a
nonprofit organization in 1997 to provide a national focal point for the
growing prevention movement. The Prevention Institute works collaboratively, engaging many different sectors and disciplines, to build momentum
for community-focused prevention strategies both locally and nationally.
For many years, I didn't like to use the abbreviation "PI" for Prevention
Institute, fearing people would think we were private investigators. Now
I welcome this association, because I realize prevention really is about
being good detectives—uncovering what fundamentally causes health and
safety problems. Like any good detective story, it's challenging, with twists
and surprises, as different types of evidence are uncovered. One thing is
certain—broadening the scope of preventive work is a job worth doing.

I became passionate about prevention when I realized it was a game changer for everyone and especially for communities where decades of disinvestment and discriminatory practices and policies have damaged neighborhood environments, diminished opportunity, and exacerbated negative health and safety impacts. Those of us who've had greater access to resources have a responsibility to recognize and shift the imbalance. Prevention is a powerful tool to support all communities, but it's designed to be of particular consequence and value to those struggling to gain fair and equal access to the fundamental conditions that support health, equity, and safety.

Throughout my career, I have deliberately directed my efforts at people directly engaged in health and related fields so that their preventive efforts would be more effective. I've always believed that as individuals, we "get" prevention and are doing our best to implement preventive measures. However, it's time, with *Prevention Diaries*, to deliver the prevention message more broadly.

Each chapter of *Prevention Diaries* presents connected elements and reflections on a particular topic—together representing elements of a single prism, or pieces of a jigsaw puzzle. This book weaves my personal stories, experiences, and reflections with critical findings from the field. The elements are intended to provide a sense of direction and opportunity and catalyze thinking for each reader. My goal, to paraphrase Einstein when he was asked to describe the theory of relativity, is to make prevention strategy "as simple as possible, but no simpler."

The sweeping community prevention successes captured throughout *Prevention Diaries* underscore the value of investing and reinvesting in prevention initiatives and the urgent need to emphasize such strategies in future thinking and policy. As more people start to understand prevention at the *community* level and engage as prevention advocates, we'll gain collective strength in pushing for the kind of community and political change our nation needs and in *pushing back* against those who have an interest in maintaining the unhealthy status quo. As this momentum snowballs, we'll advance the conditions needed to transform the current sick-care system into a true *health* system. Now is the time for all of us to work together to get it right.

INTERLUDE

CANCER

It was only after my mother died that I heard the word cancer. *Despite her symptoms and despite my growing to be a teenager and then a college student, it hadn't ever entered my consciousness that my mother had a specific illness, let alone that illness; from the time I was four, she was just "sick." On several occasions she was hospitalized and seemed near death, then a new "miracle drug" would appear and she'd be well enough to go home again. In fact, there were a few years when she was relatively healthy. In these stretches we would go to the movies, make dinner, and even go for drives to Long Island on the weekends. And then the illness would return.*

I received the call while working in a summer camp two hours from my New York City home. The head of the camp told me I needed to go home right away—packing everything, as I might not be coming back. It was a warm, breezy night as I was driven into town to the bus station. The only thing that mattered was rejoining my family and seeing my mother, perhaps for the last time.

Of course, we held out hope for a miracle. I had learned by then that "miracle drugs" meant experimental drugs. Volunteering her for drug trials wasn't always enough; often it required bribing, convincing higher-ups in the drug companies and the government that they should allow this experiment to take place. In fact, the drug she took at the end was powerful, and the next day my mother showed me how a patch of her arm was literally rotting. Each day we watched the patch get bigger and bigger. That stint in the hospital lasted twenty-one days, and she died just when the insurance ran out. "It's like she knew," my father said, "like she counted." She said many personal and important things to me in those last days, but she never said the word cancer.

[2]

UPSTREAM

RIVERS AND OCEANS

A man was walking along the bank of a river when he noticed someone drowning. He jumped in and helped the person reach the shore. Almost immediately, he saw several others in need of help. They were fully dressed, obviously not planning to go for a swim. Fortunately, there were people on the bank who could assist with the rescues. Suddenly, a woman who'd been helping began to walk upstream. "Hey, where are you going?" shouted the man. "We need you." "I'm going to see why people keep falling into the river in the first place," she replied. As it turned out, the bridge at the head of the river had a hole in it, and this was the source of the problem. The woman realized that fixing the hole would prevent people from falling into the river to begin with.

I often shared this parable when I started doing prevention work. Adapted from a poem by Joseph Malins,[1] an early prevention advocate, this story helped advance a new way of thinking, of moving metaphorically "upstream." The upstream notion has since become the seminal metaphor for quality prevention: dealing with the immediate crisis but also addressing the urgent need to reduce the number of people getting sick or injured in the first place. By moving upstream and fixing the metaphoric holes, it is possible to eliminate multiple sources of peril population-wide. The story is persuasive, and the prevention potential is powerful, but, as a society, we're not there yet. As feminist leader and journalist Gloria Steinem declared, "We are still standing on the bank of the river, rescuing people who are drowning. We have not gone to the head of the river to keep them from falling in. That is the 21st century task."[2] Doctors are trained to serve one person at a time and after maladies have arisen—"What's your complaint? What brings you here?" Their skill and dedication to saving lives is invaluable. However, their affiliated healthcare organizations have a responsibility to design effective strategies that consider both prevention and treatment—to create interventions that achieve maximum impact. Inaction in regard to prevention is not effective or wise, because it does nothing to mitigate the stream of illness coming through the door and will lead to more and more people needing to be saved.

So that's the challenge: cultivate a new way of thinking and acting *up front*, identifying clues that point to things that need improving in the environment. Nearly every illness and injury can give clues for preventing further incidents. It's incumbent on health officials and leaders to heed these clues to develop effective strategies, which are more humane and cost effective than treating patients one at a time. One at a time won't cut it—we'll never get there.[3]

AT THE PUB

When I was in London, I visited the John Snow Pub, built on the site where Dr. John Snow famously removed the handle of a water pump to prevent the pump's further spread of cholera in 1854. In addition to treating patients individually, Dr. Snow wisely decided to focus on finding the source of the problem. Studying the trends of that particular outbreak, he realized that the infected people had all drunk from one contaminated pump. Instead of simply warning locals not to drink from it, Dr. Snow removed the pump's handle, preventing new cases of cholera.

As Hippocrates put it nearly 2,000 years ago, "The function of protecting and developing health must rank even above that of restoring it."[4]

While most people in industrialized nations don't face cholera today, the lingering threat of lead exposure remains a comparable and all too common menace. Lead poisoning severely impairs the body, especially the nervous system, and is especially damaging to children, whose brains are still developing. Even low levels of exposure over time can affect children's physical and mental development, reducing the ability to concentrate, learn, and rest; slowing body growth; and causing behavioral problems. With poor diet, the effects are even greater: Blood cells absorb the lead more intensively, as the body tries to fill certain nutritional deficiencies. Eliminating lead from the body requires arduous, painful medical treatment, like chelation. Yet even after treatment, damage caused by exposure to lead is often irreversible.

Prior to the 1970s, our environment was saturated with lead in paint, gasoline, and cookware, as well as in water and soil. Thousands of children were being poisoned,[5] especially poor children, because they lived in homes where the paint was more likely to be peeling. Many also lived alongside freeways, breathing in fumes and playing in contaminated soil. In those days one could practically draw a map of the highways in the United States by looking at where lead poisoning rates were highest. Educating people about the problem was important, but education alone couldn't do much. Even for the most diligent, responsible adults, telling toddlers not to eat peeling paint or breathe lead dust or diesel fumes, particularly when their environment was permeated with these toxins, was ineffective and unrealistic. Policy changes were needed to remove lead from products and the environment.

Until 1978 lead paint was a ubiquitous presence in homes because it was bright, durable, flexible, fast-drying, and cheap. When I was repainting the exterior of my house in Oakland, I showed the painter a photo from Quito, Ecuador, where the city maintains its historic look by requiring that all homes be painted with bright blue trim. "That's the color I want," I said to the painter, who shook his head disapprovingly. "You can't do that blue," he said. "It won't stay bright since they took the lead out of paint." As I learned, the battle over lead was rooted in profit—the sale of bright, inexpensive paint—weighed against the healthy development of children.

Predictably, lobbyists in the petroleum and chemical industries and many politicians had lined up on the side of bright paint, not bright kids, even knowing the agony that lead inflicts. Once people realized that lead exposure resulted from choices that big industry and some politicians were making at the expense of children's lives, they fought back by forming coalitions and building momentum for policy change. Corporations downplayed the problem, and lobbyists tried to derail these efforts. But people didn't let up on the politicians, and eventually Congress passed sweeping legislation that removed some key sources of lead from the environment. In short, they went up the river to cut off the stream of lead.

As people's exposure decreased, the number of new cases with high blood lead levels plunged dramatically, dropping by two-thirds in just an eight-year period for children aged one to two.[6] Furthermore, the plan paid off. In addition to reducing harm, the Centers for Disease Control and Prevention calculates that every dollar spent to lower lead hazards produces a benefit ranging from $17 up to as high as $221 in reduced costs for healthcare, educational remediation, and criminal justice, among other areas.[7]

In the face of such success, it's heartbreaking and inexcusable that a quarter of a million US children—largely disadvantaged ones—continue to pay the price today, as a result of residual lead toxicity from previous generations and other exposures that aren't well regulated (as in the heartbreaking events of Flint, Michigan, in 2016). Alerted to the ongoing problems of lead, our medical providers have become much more effective in identifying lead exposures and treating them individually, on a case-by-case basis. But it takes all of us, particularly our healthcare system, to go beyond one-by-one treatment, identifying the community conditions that create exposures and insisting on policy changes to remove lead contamination at the source—*before* more damage occurs.

UPSTREAM IN THE DELTA

One of the teachers in my graduate school was Dr. Jack Geiger, whose reputation for courage and innovation preceded him. I got to know him even better when we both traveled to Cuba to investigate its health system, which was thriving despite intense poverty. A physician-advocate, Geiger had traveled to the Mississippi Delta back in 1964 on the heels of technological change that had wiped out even subsistence jobs for the area's Black sharecroppers. It was before food stamps, and hundreds of children were starving. The entire community lacked clean drinking water, which led to infections and dehydration. Geiger realized that treating people one at a time was never going to be enough. He had to develop a different approach.

He took one look at the malnourished patients at the community health clinic he founded and directed and proceeded to write prescriptions for food that could be redeemed at local grocery stores—carefully spelling out specific quantities of fruits, vegetables, or eggs. When the federal officials funding Dr. Geiger's community clinic found out about the plan, they were outraged, saying, "You can't give away food and charge it to the pharmacy budget." As Dr. Geiger recalled at a conference in 2004, "We said, 'Why not?' They said, 'Because the health center pharmacy is for drugs for treating disease.' And Jack said, 'Well, the last time I looked in the Physician's Desk Reference, the specific therapy for malnutrition was food.' " Of course, the food wasn't just for treatment; accessing nutritious fresh food is key to prevention as well. Jack saw that hunger, along with other poverty-induced conditions, had to be addressed at the root, to establish and sustain community wellness.

Geiger's colleague Dr. John Hatch soon joined him, serving as director of community health action, another name for community organizing. Eventually L.C. Dorsey, a local resident who fully understood the community context, took over operation of the clinic. Her vision and grassroots knowledge enabled her to excel both in graduate school and, more important, as the clinic leader, despite previously only having a GED. Staff at the clinic realized people didn't just need medicine for ringworm, for example, but also shoes to avoid ringworm, and thus prescriptions for shoes. They took it further, listening to members of the community and examining underlying conditions that were making people sick in the first place. Community members said, "We don't want a hand-out. We want to grow our own food—we know how." So Geiger, Hatch, and Dorsey, along with a broad team of engineers, social workers, nurses, midwives, and others, focused on helping people develop their own self-sustaining tools and skills so they could thrive independently with dignity. With resident leaders, Hatch and Dorsey led the community in digging wells, installing sanitary systems, and developing a food co-op, where more than 1,000 families grew and shared food. Geiger ordered a tractor as part of his surgical supplies. When officials reviewed his order—a rare event in his experience (and he had gambled they wouldn't)—they disallowed the tractor, but they couldn't slow community momentum.[8]

Geiger, Hatch, and Dorsey understood that the entire healthcare system lacked a focus on prevention, from the kinds of services provided most intensively to the allocation of funds. Although Geiger didn't succeed with the tractor order, his humane vision, credibility, and innovative prevention approach—as well as that of his colleagues—inspired a community-centered health movement, where their influence in speaking up about the impact of social, political, and economic factors helped broaden people's understanding of the nature of health.

Conviction and creativity like Jack Geiger's are necessary for such upstream change. The bureaucrats who questioned Dr. Geiger's approach, some of them clinicians themselves, weren't necessarily uncaring. They had a different, more limited paradigm and weren't willing to reconsider their standard approach. As Jack noted, "They recognized that this was a very different model and it would directly empower impoverished Black populations as partners in the delivery of their own health services."[9] With its roots in apartheid South Africa, where Geiger interned during medical school, this community-centered model was developed as a way of strengthening populations facing poverty conditions—addressing social and economic needs as well as medical ones.[10] An extreme apartheid regime later dismantled this vast health system in South Africa, while Geiger, on the other hand, garnered help from progressive leaders like Senator Ted Kennedy, who helped institutionalize this new approach.

The work of Geiger and Hatch, which became the prototype for community-oriented primary care in the United States, speaks to the value of pushing against the current in order to change systems and communities for the better. Remembering their work reminds me that prevention is a complex craft, combining science with artistry. The key is to engage a broader range of providers, community leaders, and public health advocates in developing this craft, as part of cultivating the skills, compassion, and vision to drive change.

THE NANNY STATE

Personal responsibility is a powerful, positive value in the United States, and it is important for health. However, the overemphasis on personal responsibility alone has, unfortunately, been systematically used as an excuse for not fully implementing prevention strategies. Our society's dominant culture generally believes individuals can—and should— change their behavior on their own, once they understand the value of healthier alternatives. We all want the freedom to decide how we choose to behave. But even if people see how behaviors lead to illness or injury and acknowledge the power of altering such behaviors, their ~~choices are~~ also influenced, and many times ~~determined, by policies, available resources, and the pervasive messages of institutions that shape their environments.~~ Thus, ~~the context in which people live has a deep impact on the range of their possible choic~~es and therefore on the illnesses and injuries that can develop as a result.

Nearly everyone values individual freedom and the opportunity for personal responsibility—the centrality of these beliefs is taken for granted in the United States—often without acknowledging the contradiction of blaming people for their choices in communities lacking healthy choices. Meanwhile, corporations spend billions on relentless marketing precisely because they're aware that they can influence individuals' choices—and take advantage of people lacking access to better options in their neighborhoods. In supermarkets, for example, people make their own choices based on what's available and affordable, yet marketers also know customers are more likely to buy what is placed near the checkout counter. In neighborhoods without supermarkets, choices are even more constrained.

~~Strong convictions about personal responsibility have been transformed to seem inherently opposed to community responsibility.~~ Almost any action taken to help people be safer or healthier has been belittled and deliberately framed as the "nanny state," shorthand for making people in the United States believe that consumer protection policies are overprotective and disrespectful of "personal choice." Corporations and lobbyists leverage the conviction about individual responsibility into opposition to implementing effective policies, claiming that individuals can make their own decisions (despite conditions that are out of individual control). In addition to making their case in the media, corporations spend billions on lobbying campaigns to block regulations that could protect people, fully knowing that health advocates can't possibly match their resources—tilting regulations, instead, in their own favor. They belittle and misrepresent almost any actions taken to help people be safer or healthier, deliberately using the dreaded nanny state frame of reference. ~~Promoting the nanny state notion has worked—it's a fear-based tactic~~ that encourages people to reject any proposed solution favoring community well-being over industry profit. ~~It has become a key barrier to advancing effective prevention.~~

In reality, community and personal responsibility are both necessary and complementary. I'm more comfortable deciding the temperature of my hotel shower because I know regulations are in place to ensure that the hotel's water system has a regulator that prevents me from unintentionally getting scalded. It's easier to skip soda in a community with clear delicious tap water. At times the nanny state arguments have been used to diminish the regulation of industry even when the general public has little control. Requiring actions to reduce lead or asthma threats is not indicative of a nanny state. A community prevention approach improves living conditions and expands the range of available options, enabling individuals who can freely access these options to make personal choices that are even more responsible. No one makes decisions in a vacuum; people are part of a community web and are responsive to the world around them. As leaders like Chip Johnson, the Republican mayor of Hernando, Mississippi, puts it, "My job is not to tell people to be healthy, but it is to create an atmosphere and opportunities for good health. If I don't have sidewalks for people to walk on or parks for our children to play in, I haven't done my job."

INTERLUDE
CONEY ISLAND

I was born in Coney Island, and even after moving to another part of New York City at age five, I returned every weekend to spend time with my grandparents. Coney Island was a special place then. It had the soft sand beaches that stretched along New York's shoreline, where families went to cool off from steamy summers in the city. The seemingly endless boardwalk ran for miles without a break. Coney Island was famous for its awe-inspiring roller coasters and the iconic parachute jump built for the 1939 New York World's Fair and later installed there. With the country's first permanent amusement park, the community had a carnival atmosphere, and it was an irresistible draw for New Yorkers looking for a getaway on the weekend—people came from all over to gawk at the "freak" shows and eat Nathan's hot dogs and French fries.

I cherished walking by myself, looking at the people and places. Even at age five, I would walk long distances down the boardwalk alone, and I loved the independence. With no streets to cross, my family didn't worry about my getting hit by a car. They didn't worry about my safety in other ways either; the environment was peaceful and the local people were attentive to me. My grandfather was universally known and respected, and most people treated me like family. Venturing down the boardwalk, I'd often sample the street food, bite-sized treats from many cultures. A precursor to fast food, it was an appealing, unique innovation. I'm not sure I appreciated that people gave me pretty much whatever I asked for, usually pizza, French fries, and frozen custard, for free. Arbes (boiled and salted chickpeas) were sold from a small pushcart, like ice cream, and they were a uniquely delicious treat (now out of fashion but might very well return). I even knew to stay away from the maple walnut ice cream—it had everything except walnuts in it—made from a combination of all the leftover flavors and strong artificial walnut flavoring, which covered up the staleness of the aging ice cream.

Coney Island was a tight-knit, off beat community. My grandfather was popular for his generosity, finding odd jobs and a bed for those who were down on their luck, despite his own poverty. People generally watched out for each other, trying to shrug off the hardships they faced. It was a place where you would use whatever odd assets you had to succeed at all costs. To the outside world, Coney Island was known as the home of drifters and freaks. The world's strongest man (he pulled a car across the beach with his teeth), the shortest man, and the two-headed woman were my companions. I thought they were the normal ones and the visitors were the odd ones. Coming to escape their mundane existence, visitors readily entered a world of "tricks and funny mirrors." They gawked and laughed at the members of the freak shows for 25 cents a view and, as far as my young eyes could see, the freaks weren't self-conscious or angry about it. I never questioned these norms, which were in no way seen as immoral or disrespectful—exploitation was the expectation. Separating willing tourists from their money helped sustain the neighborhood. I imagined it as a Robin Hood story, where the poor cast offs were kept afloat by fleecing the affluent visitors.

The strongest man was nearly seventy, an unimaginable age to me when I turned five. He sold his strength via an elixir—a special formula he promised would make anyone "almost as strong" as he was. My parents remembered that he had won an Olympic gold medal, and while they stood at the edge of the crowd and marveled at the way he pulled the car, they were quick to caution that there were no elixirs. Turning down the shortest man, who was vending the product, my parents told me that the only thing the elixir would accomplish was to keep the two of them fed. They said this was a good thing and that plenty of tourists would help them achieve this goal.

The shortest man was four feet tall and lived in a very small, cheap, shoddily sparsely furnished room that my grandparents rented out for extra income. He was known for his TV commercials during the dawn of television. In the commercials, he posed as a hotel barker, at a time when a fancy hotel might have had a "midget," as they were then called. Dressed in a jester's suit, he walked *through the lobby announcing telephone calls, among other things, since there were no room phones then. He was famous for his tobacco commercial, "Call for Philip Morris," a clever play on words. I liked visiting with him and was proud when I saw his ads on TV. One weekend when I came to my grandparents, I learned he had "moved out." I was told "lung cancer." I was too young to think about the irony and tragedy of this.*

I loved the Coney Island spirit, but since then, the good-natured manipulations of Coney Island have been co-opted, corrupted, and exaggerated in our country. Street food became fast food and went from being an occasional treat to a daily norm cloaked in "new and improved" and "heart healthy" labels. Rather than going of their own free will to a unique place for weekend entertainment, where deception was understood to be part of the climate, people are now faced with daily deception for profit, as ads for unhealthy products fleece not only our pocketbooks but also damage our well-being. While the freaks wooed the willing with elixirs to seek a living, today's pharmaceuticals stalk the vulnerable with elixirs with the goal of making a massive profit. Both offered the promise of long life, but buyers beware—if you can.

[3]

IT'S THE ENVIRONMENT

LUNCH WITH THE TOBACCO LOBBYIST

The head lobbyist for the tobacco industry leaned forward in his chair. He was dapper in a dark suit, and he was unfazed as rings of smoke wafted from neighboring tables in the swank restaurant where we were meeting; perhaps he even liked it. I marveled at his lavish words of praise for my prevention efforts, which he, to my surprise, knew a lot about. (This was pre-Internet, so his research was even more impressive.)

It was 1984. Only a few days before this lunch, I had convened a coalition to propose the first countywide, multicity regulations banning smoking in restaurants, workplaces, and other public spaces. That first coalition meeting was deliberately small, with only the local leadership from the American Heart Association, American Lung Association, and American Cancer Society and me. At the time I was head of the prevention program for Contra Costa, a county in northern California. Our group's collaborative effort marked a shift for these health organizations, which generally competed with one another for funds. In the past, they had focused on dealing with the aftermath of their respective ailments, funneling funds into research, services for the afflicted, and treatment. But what if it were possible to stop the diseases before they started? The scientific verdict was in, confirming that tobacco killed; yet individuals trying to quit or not start faced a barrage of well-financed, emotionally charged messages from the tobacco industry: "You've Come a Long Way, Baby"; "Camel: Where a Man Belongs."[1]

Together, the coalition was plotting how to convince each of the 18 city councils in Contra Costa to sign onto our proposed smoking ban. We had decided on early-morning meetings at a local diner to allow the doctors in our group to participate before going to their medical practices. It wasn't an easy task: cities rarely legislated health then, and they certainly didn't think tobacco was an issue that pertained to them. But the personal connections and credibility of both the physicians and the donors who supported these health organizations (and contributed to local political campaigns) turned out to be key.

Within 24 hours of that first meeting, the tobacco industry's head lobbyist had contacted me and suggested lunch. He immediately steered the conversation from tobacco to our county's car-seat initiative, on which he appeared well versed. He smiled and asked, "Larry, how many car seats do you want?" I fumbled. I thought, we could use an additional 40 to distribute locally; it could encourage those with limited resources to start using car seats. But in preparation for the meeting, a colleague had advised me to multiply all numbers by 10 when speaking to any lobbyist, so I was thinking 400. In my confusion, I found myself suddenly adding another zero and suggested 4,000. He didn't blink. Then our conversation turned to employment opportunities for me in the tobacco industry.

"Look, I'll triple your salary," he offered. The proposal was that I would still work on tobacco prevention but for them and—this was important to him—on subjects not involving tobacco policy.

"Larry, we're not against telling people that smoking is unhealthy," he told me. "We'll even publish a book warning people about the dangers of smoking—with your name as author engraved in gold letters on the cover!" I demurred, and I thought about my mother. Under other circumstances, she would have been proud to see my name in gold letters. But she had died of cancer (in no way related to tobacco), and the idea that someone could consciously inflict cancer on anyone was jarring, even chilling. The lobbyist misunderstood my pensiveness.

"Anything you want. You name it," he continued. Then lowering his voice, he added, "We just want to stay away from policy."

"You said you're a parent, right?" I asked him.

"Yes, my son is 10," he replied, welcoming the way the conversation seemed to have turned.

I looked at him hard before saying, "How do you explain to your son why you're encouraging people to die from cancer?"

The lunch was over.

Our group's consistent countywide measure (across 18 cities) was arguably the most important of the early smoking-prevention legislation. Similar measures had previously been passed in San Francisco and Berkeley—both liberal cities, which led to their bans' dismissals as "fringe"—and in Minnesota, which had passed a state-wide clean air act. (The Minnesota effort, while quite significant in its statewide scope, didn't require any specific percentages of public establishments to be nonsmoking, just that accommodation for nonsmokers exist alongside accommodation for smokers.) Our Contra Costa legislation passed overwhelmingly in every setting—rural, suburban, and urban—in politically diverse and relatively conservative Contra Costa County, California, making it the most sweeping and surprising legislation of its kind. It was supported by a coalition of nonprofits, government, and local residents, and its specific language gave little room for evasion or selective uptake across the county. Our growing movement quickly built momentum and national attention, expanding beyond restaurants and government service sites to focus on airline flights, workplaces, public spaces, and then even removal of cigarettes from vending machines. As Mark Pertschuk, head of Americans for Nonsmokers' Rights, put it, "Without victories like Contra Costa County, we would not have won the airline smoking ban campaign in the late 1980s. It was the grassroots revolution."[2] He estimates the Contra Costa effort helped lead to 200 other local ordinances against smoking.

By the time big tobacco reached settlement agreements with states across the country more than a decade later, hundreds of communities had authorized local smoke-free ordinances. The power to transform the environment came because we were building a movement and prompting a new set of expectations and standards for what was desirable and acceptable. Restrictions that appeared minor were significant enough to start the ball rolling in altering tobacco consumption patterns, which accelerated the shift in social norms. It was clear that people increasingly understood the associated health risks, and that galvanized the political will to fight back. Industry and lobbyists were unable to stop the tide as regulations helped alter smoking norms, and the change in norms led to stepped-up policy efforts.

Negative health impacts fell correspondingly. The idea of *not smoking* seemed odd to many at first, but it was precisely this oddity that prompted people to rethink their habits and expectations. Before, nonsmokers were used to stepping outside in the rain to get a breath of fresh air. Suddenly, it was the smokers who had to go outside. This shift also sent a strong message about the dangers of inhaling secondhand smoke. By providing an alternative to traditional ways of thinking, the early ordinances got people thinking about whether they wanted to inhale smoke as they ate dinner or flew on an airplane.

If this campaign had been mounted now, it would have been labeled part of the "nanny state." But, needless to say, our efforts actually expanded options, creating the possibility of flying and eating out without inhaling smoke. They helped people see that smoke in their environment wasn't a fact they had to accept as normal. One of the greatest accomplishments of prevention occurs when people no longer view unhealthy, unsafe norms as inevitable; instead, they begin to insist that communities, industries, and leaders not deliberately allow the conditions that unnecessarily harm people.

TENNESSEE AS THE INNOVATOR IN CAR SEAT SAFETY

Dr. Bob Sanders is the Tennessee pediatrician who promoted the nation's first car seat law. Correct use of a car seat doubles a child's likelihood of surviving a car crash uninjured, but, despite broad awareness, less than 25 percent of young children rode in car seats prior to the law's passage in Tennessee in 1977. Despite the obvious benefits, Dr. Sanders encountered a lot of opposition in his home state when he fought for the law. In fact, he told me that the state director of a major national medical association testified that "authorizing this as law would take away parents' God-given right to make decisions for their own children."

Sanders was steadfast in his belief that families needed stronger laws to support them in changing habitual ways of thinking and behaving. He persevered in building the political will to make these changes law, largely through "back-fence diplomacy"—reaching out to legislators he and his wife, Pat, already knew.[3] Wisely, they made it a very personal crusade, where it was clear that real people—real children—were at stake. Once the legislation passed, just like the local tobacco laws, it ignited similar laws across the country. By now, these laws have kept thousands of children alive and countless more saved from serious injuries.[4] Most parents now are grateful for this type of legislation, and nearly 100 percent of infants ride in car seats.

Sanders's law also catalyzed other supportive changes for infants and children. Hospital staff began escorting parents to their cars to ensure safe transport for newborns, which enhanced the likelihood of parents starting to use the seats regularly. In fact, hospitals would not release newborns until they were in a proper car seat. If parents contested, they had to acknowledge they were acting against medical advice, just as if they were taking their child home with a dangerously high fever. Communities responded with training programs, where law enforcement and volunteers taught parents how to properly install the seats and buckle children in. Communities also developed programs to distribute car seats to parents with low incomes. In California, we use the revenue from car seat traffic stops to fund this, which helps police be more comfortable making the stops, knowing the fines serve to further protect children. Most parents also found it was easier for them to travel with children in car seats.

Today car seats are so ingrained in the culture of child-raising that they pass the "prevention take-back" test: even if the legislation were to change back now, most people would probably continue to use car seats because the law established a new norm, and this norm then changed the behaviors in more responsible and health-promoting ways. When I talk about this example now, people say, "It was easy with car seats, because their value is so obvious." Talking with Bob and Pat Sanders, it's clear that it was only easy in retrospect.

TAKING TWO STEPS TO PREVENTION

People are often shocked to hear that researchers have found 70 percent of illnesses and injuries are due to human behavior and the environments we live in, versus only 10 percent from lack of medical care (the remaining

20 percent are attributed to genetics). Sometimes it's hard to see how the things we do daily and the beliefs we take for granted can have such a large influence on our health and safety. It's even more difficult to recognize how the social and physical environments affect both our behavior and well-being.

To help people identify these broader influences and determine how to advance health and safety, the Prevention Institute introduced the concept of Taking Two Steps to Prevention. We explain first how medical conditions are influenced by our behavior, then how behaviors are largely determined by factors in our community and environment. Starting with a medical condition (say, type 2 diabetes), we first look for clues that reveal the behavior or exposure that contributed to it (e.g., lack of physical activity). Then we identify community conditions that shaped the behavior (e.g., lack of safe places to be active and play, no sidewalks or infrastructure for walking and biking, overdependence on driving as our means of transportation). It really is a detective story. As a society, the United States collectively deludes itself into thinking that people are simply dying prematurely of natural causes, when any good detective could identify and intercept the perpetrators.

Around the time my prevention work began, two health researchers, Drs. Mike McGinnis and Bill Foege, coined the term *actual causes*. The term referred to the connection between a handful of relatively common behaviors and exposures that determine how likely we are to suffer the leading causes of death, illness, and injury. *Do we smoke? Do we eat well? Do we wear a seat belt and put seat belts on our kids? Do we own or carry a gun? Are we exposed to toxins? How much do we drink? Are we physically active?* Their choice of the term *actual causes* helped people understand that these underlying influences shape the likelihood of whether they will be injured or become ill.

Further, the *actual causes* are shaped by the policies, practices, and norms we see in our neighborhoods, workplaces, and schools. *Do we live in neighborhoods with access to healthy food? Is it served in the schools, or is the healthy food lacking entirely?* Recognizing the underlying influence of our environments is extremely important, because it makes it clear that people do not have to get sick or injured so frequently. It's not just a question of fate, lack of personal responsibility, or inherently bad decision-making on the part of individuals. ~~Personal responsibility and community conditions~~ ~~go hand in hand.~~

Once people understand that their behaviors impact their health and safety, they can—and do—make better decisions, if the environment supports their efforts toward healthier behaviors. At the time I started focusing on no-smoking laws, the scientific evidence linking chronic smoking with lung cancer was still emerging, even though it's taken for granted today. Many people were even more surprised and skeptical about the effects of secondhand smoke, since smoke was accepted as a natural part of the indoor environment back then. Understanding these links and realizing that quitting reduces the risk, both for users and bystanders, were important first steps. Creating smoke-free environments made it possible for people to quit successfully.

For Dr. John Snow, reducing cholera was relatively easy: don't just warn people the water is risky—identify and disable the pump at the source. Many conditions are more complex, but most of the forces that influence them have already been identified. Taking the appropriate action based on what has been learned can save many lives. This is exactly what a good healthcare provider does: track back from the clinical concern, uncover the cause of the problem, and determine the right treatment to arrest it. A preventionist's approach is similar.

When I do training on Two Steps to Prevention, I show photos to guide people in how to do prevention detective work. First, I might show a photo of a serious car crash and ask the audience what is needed in response to the crash. People immediately focus on the need for swift, high-quality medical care. Next, taking the first step, I reveal evidence of

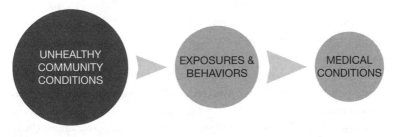

Figure 1 Trajectory of Health Inequity

what caused the crash, showing a picture of two people drinking heavily and laughing. When people see this, it shifts their frame of mind, and they start thinking about ways to solve the underlying problem of drinking and driving. They start to realize the behavior triggered the need for medical care; the crash was not an "accident."

Taking the second step reveals how our environments and norms reinforce this risky behavior in so many ways. I show a photo a staff member took of a storefront sign that says, "Drive-in liquor." It's not a mystery. Many factors in our environment foster this behavior—widespread advertisements promoting alcohol use as glamorous, sexy, and fulfilling; social norms condoning alcohol use; easy access for youth; peer pressure; and an emphasis on driving in our culture, with a lack of viable public transportation. Every time I walk through an airport I see signs pointing to defibrillators—wisely ready to revive someone suffering from a heart attack—though the entire airport corridor smells of fried chicken, burgers, and, most notably, cinnamon rolls (with additional aroma pumped out of vents to entice more purchasing). So airports are not only prepared for heart attacks; they promote them.

These links probably seem obvious, yet the United States is still putting nearly all of its healthcare resources into after-the-fact clinical care, instead of applying a conceptual understanding of the underlying influences.

MADD

Sometimes it takes a tragedy for us to change our expectations and practices. When Candy Lightner's thirteen-year-old daughter, Cari, was killed by a drunk driver in 1980, Candy understandably focused her rage on the irresponsible person behind the wheel. Despite his multiple arrests for drinking and driving, the driver hadn't served any jail time, and his sentence of two years for Cari's death was predictably light. In those days, it was socially acceptable to drive home after a night of heavy drinking. Comedians lampooned it, and the popular movie *Arthur* turned the escapades of the "happy drunk" into a standing joke. I grew up watching *Topper,* a highly rated TV show featuring a talking St. Bernard that loved to drink Scotch from his bowl. While of course there was a lack of reality to a show about a dog, it nevertheless aligned with attitudes that drinking was mostly a laughing matter.

Candy got angry every time she saw things like this. For her, it wasn't a conceptual exercise to take two steps to prevention: it was a visceral response to an environment that encouraged reckless behavior and led to deaths like Cari's. People received information warning them about drinking and driving, but the deck was stacked against that information affecting their behavior. Around the time that Cari was killed, I went to an alcohol prevention meeting, where a dentist said he'd been arrested twenty-three times for drunk driving but never had to serve jail time. He didn't receive meaningful treatment services either. It was handled as if it weren't likely to happen again—though it predictably was. As a well-respected professional, he was granted continual leniency *until he eventually hurt someone.* The lack of intervention revealed society's norm of not taking this issue seriously—and not thinking about prevention as a strategy—until it was too late.

Candy catalyzed the movement for change. She started with the court system, which had failed to shape norms with laws that repudiated drunk driving. Despite her persuasiveness and poignant story, Candy realized she alone couldn't accomplish broad change. She reached out to other victims through classified ads. Together, they formed Mothers Against Drunk Driving: MADD—a brilliant acronym reinforcing the passionate commitment to preventive change.

They were fighting the alcohol industry, whose words said, "Don't drink and drive" but whose actions focused on the opposite outcome—for example, marketing alcohol in gas stations. Profiting from heavy drinking in our car-dependent society, the alcohol industry takes drunk-driving deaths (and any other harmful impacts of alcohol use) as collateral damage. MADD partnered with insurance companies and banks to finance a counterattack. Car rental companies and carmakers eventually joined ranks. Candy reached out to youth to engage them in reducing underage drinking and build their leadership. This helped counter the effects of ads targeting them with the message that drinking would make them happier, more grown up, and more likely to achieve sexual conquests. Gaining momentum, MADD catalyzed others to act.

One of my favorite youth-led efforts was "Friday Night Live," pioneered by Dr. Jim Kooler. The program educated high school students about risks of alcohol and driving. Its centerpiece was a teen-staffed phone line that was available to the public. Anyone who had had too much to drink could call for a safe ride home, no questions asked. While originally created to reduce car crashes, this service also served as a powerful initiative against many of the crimes associated with drinking, particularly helping young women to avoid situations where they were at risk for sexual violence.

Advocates also targeted venues serving alcohol, where they trained bartenders and wait staff to limit patrons' alcohol intake and to encourage intoxicated patrons to not drive home. (It's interesting to note that the alcohol industry actually co-opted the idea of the designated driver and developed a sophisticated campaign that put all the responsibility on individuals and only discouraged drinking for the one person who would be driving). Further efforts led to the elimination of alcohol sales in the fourth quarter or late innings of sporting events, altering practices across the country. Major policy changes followed: banning driving with an open alcohol container; lowering the legal blood alcohol content for driving; and, perhaps most important, creating a higher uniform drinking age across the United States.

As with the anti-tobacco movement, the strategies and controversies led to extensive media coverage—far more than with a stand-alone informational campaign—and the media repeatedly gave people facts about the risks of drinking. However, MADD never said that alcohol itself had to be eliminated. Of course, as long as alcohol is available, there will be excesses that result not only in DUIs but also in violence and medical concerns like cirrhosis. Yet fewer people in the United States today indulge in unhealthy drinking behaviors, as compared to thirty years ago,[5] and the movement has prevented tens of thousands of unnecessary deaths.[6]

EVERY LEVEL AT ONCE: THE SPECTRUM OF PREVENTION

By looking at the emerging success of different prevention efforts, patterns became evident. I realized that we had to encourage change in the working

methods of practitioners and reposition education as an importar
an all-inclusive strategy, rather than as a stand-alone effort. At t_
I discovered Dr. Marshall Swift's comprehensive approach to helping
people with developmental disabilities return to the community setting.[7]
Swift found reintegration was far more successful when institutions such
as community centers, libraries, and grocery stores had accommodating
practices and policies. Inspired by this multifaceted approach and model,
I created a framework called the Spectrum of Prevention,[8] which practitioners and communities have used as a tool for shaping a comprehensive
approach.

The Spectrum of Prevention helps communities build solutions on six
levels simultaneously: individual skills, community education, provider
training, collaboration, organizational practice, and policy. It is designed
to engage a variety of stakeholders who, by working together, can shape a
comprehensive strategy that meets the needs of *all* community members.
With each *spectrum* level of activity supporting the other five, communities can create a constellation of effective improvements with deep, lasting
health and societal impacts. MADD was a prime example of the Spectrum
in action; the movement to encourage breastfeeding was another.

wow

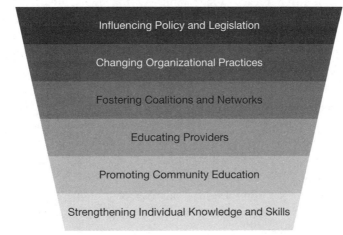

THE SPECTRUM OF PREVENTION

Influencing Policy and Legislation

Changing Organizational Practices

Fostering Coalitions and Networks

Educating Providers

Promoting Community Education

Strengthening Individual Knowledge and Skills

Figure 2 The Spectrum of Prevention

Recently, while seeking a local late-night restaurant in my travels, I ended up reading a discussion blog on Zagat, the popular restaurant guide. The topic of the day was whether women should be allowed to breastfeed in restaurants. One person responded, "Of course," but another said, "Well, it's okay perhaps in a fast food restaurant, but I wouldn't want to see it in a more formal setting." One mother of a teenager asked, "If a mother breastfed at a nearby table, what would I tell my son she was doing?"

What could be more natural than breastfeeding? It's ideal for the physical and mental health of babies and moms and is built-in effective prevention. Breastfeeding lowers risk of infection in babies, improves children's ability to learn, strengthens immunity, and reduces heart disease and diabetes. Breastfeeding also decreases the risk of ovarian cancer for mothers. Studies also show that supporting breastfeeding can lead to significant cost savings—an estimated $13 billion annually in the United State.[9] Until the early 1900s, nearly all babies were breastfed, primarily by their mothers. Some wealthy families relied on wet nurses—presumably not noticing or caring about—the oppressive contradictions of this.

Breastfeeding rates in the United States dropped precipitously around the time that corporations developed infant formula, marketing it as a convenient, high-status alternative to breastfeeding. The push away from breastfeeding also stemmed from the increasing sexualization of women in broadcast media, making it seem inappropriate for a woman to bare her breast in public. Women were even arrested or fined in some states for doing so.[10] Additionally, as more women entered the workforce, they increasingly turned to formula in response to both the stigma of breastfeeding in public and the prolonged separation from their infants.[11]

Prior to the 1970s, studies show that most women in the United States entered the hospital planning to breastfeed but were undermined along the way. Formula manufacturers provided doctors with free samples and hosted fancy receptions and "educational events" at medical conferences to cultivate good will. They also worked to ensure that nurseries in hospitals provided formula to new moms instead of offering help with breastfeeding, creating a culture of barriers too great for even the most determined mothers.

The most insidious marketing was not in the United States but in the developing world, particularly Africa and Latin America, where corporate representatives and aggressive advertising campaigns convinced mothers that formula was a healthier alternative to breast milk. Since these campaigns occurred partly in markets of scarce financial resources and inconsistent water supplies, countless babies died when they became unnecessarily dependent on formula and their mothers had ceased to produce milk.

In the United States, there's been a slow upward trend in breastfeeding since around 1970, with advocates leading comprehensive efforts to encourage its revival. Awareness of the issue has been increasing, in part, due to the outrage at international marketing campaigns. However, even as these rates increase, they change the least in low-income communities, in part because of a lack of infrastructure to support mothers and breastfeeding.

Although it wasn't explicit, the movement followed strategies delineated across the Spectrum of Prevention, each building on the other. There were initiatives to place coaches into hospitals right from the start, so women were supported in strengthening their individual knowledge and skill with breastfeeding; leaders fostered positive word of mouth to widely promote community education about the value of breastfeeding; and my favorite media-oriented event was when friends in Berkeley, California, entered the *Guinness Book of World Records* by being part of the largest group of breastfeeding moms in history.

With more nursing mothers in the workforce, US and worldwide coalitions such as La Leche League led the effort to apply pressure on large companies to change their practices—for example, extending maternity leave and providing better lactation support for nursing women while on the job. They urged hospitals to disassociate from formula marketers and align themselves with baby-friendly international coalitions, such as the International Baby Food Action Network, which influences policy on breastfeeding and formula from the local level on up to the World Health Organization. Social norms began to shift. Breastfeeding rates started to rise, and organizations such as ours started to *take it for granted* that practices like these should be implemented. Coalitions succeeded in passing national and state regulations, permitting women to breastfeed on air-planes and in other public places. As state law in Massachusetts essentially says, "Anywhere it's legal to have a young child, it's legal to breastfeed."[12]

So we've learned: a comprehensive approach to prevention, where equitable change is simultaneously enacted across all systems and norms, helps move "beyond brochures"—improving health and safety broadly and justly and saving countless lives.

[4]

WE BUILD OUR ENVIRONMENT, AND THEN IT BUILDS US

LOSING THE RED CAR

When I was invited to do injury prevention training across Hawaii, I had the opportunity to explore the beauty of the islands in my leisure time. After snorkeling one day, I managed to get an earache; fortunately, there is a medication to treat it, shrewdly named Swimmer's Ear. Arriving at midnight at my destination, Kona Kailua, I drove straight to the pharmacy and was relieved to find it was open and stocked with this medication.

But my good spirits didn't last long. When I exited the pharmacy, I realized that my car was gone. As I looked around the virtually empty lot, I didn't see a single red car. I couldn't believe it. I'd left everything in that car—my clothes, my work, the lei I had been given as a thank you for my previous talk, even the name and directions to my hotel. For a second, I thought there might have been another parking lot, but there wasn't. Bewildered, I kept walking in circles, as though my car would magically reappear.

Then I spotted a purple car with a lei draped around the mirror. Approaching it, I saw a few things on the seat that looked familiar. It wasn't my red car, but when I tried the key, it opened.

Unimaginable—how could my car have changed colors? It turns out Hawaii is home to one of the world's most prominent astronomical research observatories, and to maintain the visibility of distant stars, the observatory requires use of only low-level yellow sodium vapor bulbs in the vicinity. This yellow cast from the parking lot lights changed my red car to purple.

Now, of course, I know that color isn't fixed. Humans see it based on lenses, cones, and reflections, and as they shift, so do perceptions of color. But science had little to do with my outlook while standing in that parking lot at midnight; I expected to find my car as I thought I had left it five minutes earlier. It didn't even occur to me to look for a car that wasn't red.

Similarly, we take many aspects of our community surroundings for granted, not seeing the possibilities for how they could be different. Elements in our day-to-day environment affect our experience in critical ways, yet their effect and our ability to alter them, thus changing the effect, often go unnoticed.

I forgot all about this effect until I joined my colleague at a conference in Washington, DC, where we were both speakers. Mark Fenton is a walkability expert, professor at Tufts University, previous editor of *Walking* magazine, and host of the PBS program *America's Walking*. When Fenton gives a speech, he goes outside the conference room. He encourages conference attendees to join him first for an early morning walk around the neighborhood. I am not an early riser, but having enjoyed Fenton's strolls elsewhere around the country, on this particular morning I grabbed a cup of strong coffee and went to meet him. A group of conference attendees was waiting in front of the hotel in the very quiet pretraffic dawn.

We were staying right outside DC city limits, near National Airport and along the Chesapeake. First we headed to the path along the river, where we could hear the birds and the gentle movement of the water. We noted how the pathway was ideal not only for pedestrians but also for bicyclists, baby carriages, and wheelchairs. There were no crossings, and the pathway was relatively flat. It was tranquil, and I could practically walk with my eyes closed, to better listen, feel the air, and smell the flowers. Suddenly, an airplane flew by, low and loud; we were in the airport-landing path. Each time a plane went by, it was a complete transformation from serene to unpleasant. I wondered how the birds experienced it—were they disrupted, oblivious, or in-between? Clearly the airport's decision that flight paths would follow the river changed the entire experience. When it became quiet again, I appreciated the stillness even more, although it took a couple of minutes before I could again hear the subtler sounds. From there we made our way to the nearby main street, where walking required more focus. There weren't a lot of vehicles,

but they sped by, and although each intersection had pedestrian crossings, we quickly realized that cars and trucks frequently ignored them.
Someone noticed certain crosswalks had no curb cuts, which would be
an obstacle for wheelchairs or baby carriages. The road we now strode on
was very wide, dominating our experience, with closed office buildings at
our side and little charm. After a few more blocks, we eased onto a smaller
street, where some of the shuttered cafes had left their chairs and tables
out. The store windows were colorful and interesting. At one café, even
though it was closed, we noted the residual smell of coffee, and that made
me happy.

Fenton helped us see how the small neighborhood street had been
redesigned to be different than it once was, and later, when he spoke,
he showed plans of how the thoroughfare could become more attractive, safer, and cleaner too. We sat at tables together and discussed other
options we could envision. I realized my experience changed dramatically
based on the surroundings where we walked. I found it is not only colors
we perceive as fixed: we design and build our roads, houses, and factories
and then take for granted that it's just how they are.

Someone pointed out that streets represent the largest collection of
real estate most cities own and control.

"Well," I said, "that sounds interesting but irrelevant."

"Not irrelevant at all," Fenton said, and he proceeded to show sketches
of a narrower street with people mingling, chatting, sipping coffee, and
shopping. In cases where drab factories or billboards lined the street, he
replaced them with clever and inspiring murals.

Not irrelevant at all.

REDESIGNING OUR DECISIONS

Roads, houses, and parks are part of what some call the *built environment.*
This term refers to everything we design and construct, including homes,
schools, offices, factories, shopping malls, recreation centers, and theaters.
The streets and open spaces that connect these places are also part of the
built environment. Just as air and water—what's traditionally thought of
as *the environment*—impact our health, so does the built environment.

The location of roadways, the design of our schools, and the distance between workplaces and homes all affect our physical, mental, and social well-being.

When we design our physical structures and open spaces, we're defining their relationship to the community environment. That means reconsidering our surroundings in the same way I was forced to contemplate how my red car had changed to purple. Though it's hard to do, I try to think of our entire environment, both natural and built, as a palette. The "colors" we choose and where we place them determine how pleasing the entire design will be—and with it, how healthy we will be when we live in it. As Winston Churchill put it, "We shape our buildings, and afterwards our buildings shape us."[1]

Design decisions can serve as a powerful symbol of our community's values. For example, when Jimmy Carter installed solar panels on the roof of the White House, he demonstrated to the United States that the search for renewable energy was a priority for his administration and for the future of the country. When Ronald Reagan took them down, many felt that it signaled his commitment to our continued dependence on oil and coal instead. Then Barack Obama reinstated solar panels on the East Wing of the White House during his presidency.

The precise benefits of a health-encouraging built environment are an emerging and complex area of public health research. What is generally accepted is that the arc of US innovation has brought about urban and suburban development since the 1960s that runs counter to what's good for us: roads and highways have been emphasized over community assets such as parks, sidewalks, and bicycle lanes. The built environment influences how physically active we are or how sedentary;[2] how easily we can purchase and grow fresh, healthy food in our neighborhoods;[3,4] how safely our children can walk or bike to school;[5] whether families can live in housing that is affordable and free of industrial and road pollution.[6] The mission of public health in the twenty-first century, according to an Institute of Medicine committee comprised of our nation's top scientists and health professionals, is to assure conditions in which people can be healthy.[7] The built environment is a key channel which we do this.

THE END OF PARKING METERS

The parking meter is among the most annoying inventions of modern life, one that always makes me realize that my personal dependence on my car is very much a decision—and confirming that it's one I should reconsider. When I think about all the health and safety problems brought on by the US addiction to driving, I have to wonder, what if we "lost" our cars more often and "found" our walking legs? Maybe when I lost my car in Hawaii, I should have let it go—a sign that it was time to move on from cars.

In 2005 a group of activists reimagined the environment by feeding a single meter—and turning a parking space into a miniature park for two hours.[8,9] They filled the area with sod, a bench, and a tree, effectively making it a place of rest and relaxation within the city. In doing so, they showed that the public space at the edge of sidewalks is valuable real estate in terms of its capacity to satisfy human needs—not car needs. News of this small, single statement spread, blossoming into an annual event called PARK(ing) Day, where residents all over the world turn metered spaces into recreational areas. The concept has since expanded, with participants taking over parking spaces to plant urban gardens, conduct ecology demonstrations, and offer bike-repair services on a designated day each September.

Similar creative thinking has inspired a growing national interest in "parklets," where businesses, schools, and community organizations reclaim parking spaces or vacant plots of land for ongoing use as public gathering places.[10] Each has a unique "personality," with seating ranging from colorful café chairs to hand-hewn benches with fragrant planters. Bike racks, sculptures, and other forms of community art are woven into the mix of building materials and nature.[11] Public spaces like these foster not just health but a sense of belonging in one's community.[12]

There are many other parklet purposes. I visited San Francisco's Ciencia Pública: Agua (Public Science: Water)[13] parklet, where students and community members learn about sustainable water use and harvest free edible plants. This is a National Science Foundation project to increase informal science and technology learning and careers among populations that haven't had access to this type of learning. Located in front of a Spanish immersion school, this parklet extends the campus and curriculum, which local residents helped design. While the community environment strongly affects children's health and safety, youth usually have very little control of their surroundings. However, youth and their families have had a strong voice in shaping this project, now a prototype for a national model. The parklet movement has also led to urban "mini-farms," with people cultivating healthy foods in public gardens. Successful urban mini-farming increases access to fresh produce in low-income neighborhoods; enhances safety, trust, and community bonding; and provides residents with new economic opportunities in otherwise underutilized spaces.

WILD RAVINES, LUSH MEADOWS, AND WOOD-FILLED WORK SPACE

Design affects our mood and thus our health. It's intuitive—and well researched—that trees and greenery lift our moods, but until Frederick Law Olmsted came along in the second half of the nineteenth century,[14] most outdoor design was limited to cemeteries, where people would picnic near family graves. Olmsted promoted the idea that people would be happier, healthier, and more drawn to living in urban areas if they had daily access to beautiful parks for physical and social enjoyment.[15] He designed urban parks around the country—including New York's iconic Central Park—with both calming and stimulating experiences that eased the stress of city living. He's now known as the father of US landscape architecture, and, in numerous cities, his parks are among the landmarks of which residents are proud.

Olmsted considered Brooklyn's Prospect Park his masterpiece. His design concept there allowed people to immerse themselves in nature, exploring wild ravines, lush meadows, and grand esplanades. Ironically, he built it because he was dissatisfied with Central Park, feeling that the roadways cutting through it damaged its tranquility. When I was growing up near Prospect Park, not many people even knew what it had to offer, since it was far too dangerous for wandering. I'd only go there with my parents, and only to certain parts. Drug dealers had taken over the kids' carousel. Muggings were frequent, and people occasionally were shot. Then, in 1980, Tupper Thomas, a Minnesota transplant, began renovating the park.[16] Reaching out broadly, she formed the Prospect Park Alliance, a public–private partnership whose biggest challenge at first was getting people to use the park. They wisely lured dog owners by setting aside space for an off-leash dog area. As the big dogs and their owners started to repopulate the park, it became a safer, more desirable destination, drawing more people. Now more than 9 million annual visitors enjoy the entire park's meadows, rivers, waterfalls, lake, and boathouse—a calm respite from city life.[17]

My work space in Oakland, California, influences my sense of well-being and productivity each day, and I imagine that's true for everyone. Most mornings, walking into Prevention Institute's office building makes me feel happy. A few years back, we relocated in order to accommodate our organization's growth. Finding a property in central or downtown Oakland was part of our ongoing commitment to invest in the city's redevelopment. We didn't want to be part of the gentrification that prices long-standing residents or businesses out of their communities, replacing them and their cultures with "neighborhood improvements." So we selected an unoccupied former industrial site in an area that has a vibrant history.

We redesigned the space to emphasize openness and light. Instead of using modern building materials, which can harm health, we kept the original wood floors, ceilings, and skylights. The "walls" are recycled windows with vintage frames, which create a village-like experience that harmonizes with the neighborhood's emerging mix of heavier industry, live–work spaces, artists' lofts, cafes, and farmers' markets. We designed open stairwells, flexible workspaces, and large communal gathering areas to encourage fluid interactions and creativity. A rooftop garden is our own green space, and the view gives us a sense of our place in the community. We frequently eat or hold meetings there in the natural sunlight. In general, PI staff don't have the eyestrain, the headaches, and the dullness that can come with the typical office setup; employees and visitors report feeling inspired and engaged. As the design encourages interactions between people, it enhances understanding of one another's work.

SOCIAL POLICY IN CONCRETE

Concerned about lagging productivity, factory owners in nineteenth-century London wanted to know why so many workers were getting sick. Many blamed it on poor people, believing that "sickness came from the package of dirty habits, dirty houses, and sin," as Dr. Tom Farley, former New York health commissioner, reported in his book, *Prescription for a Healthy Nation.*[18] Health leaders at the time, however, identified over-crowded housing as the true culprit. People can't be packed into tene-ments, with little hygiene and no hot water, and *not* have diseases spread. Sure enough, expanding access to clean water and good sanitation sys-tems and plumbing in London slashed rates of illness, including cholera. Amazingly, this was done before there was a complete understanding of germs. As Farley wrote, "What may have been the greatest improvement in population health was brought about without any successful cures for any disease."[19]

Dr. Dick Jackson was one of the first to connect the built environ-ment with many of today's chronic physical and psychological conditions. As Jackson and his colleagues Howard Frumkin and Lawrence Frank describe, "The modern America of obesity, inactivity, depression, and loss of community has not 'happened' to us. We legislated, subsidized, and planned it this way."[20] Simply put, Jackson says, "The built environ-ment is social policy in concrete."[21] Nowhere is this reflected more starkly and more disappointingly than in some low-income communities of color where historical and persistent disinvestment correlates with high rates of chronic disease and injury. Instead of applying our learning to signifi-cantly improve all communities, the knowledge and policy efforts have been used destructively.

THE AIR-CONDITIONED NIGHTMARE

For several generations, many people chased the "American dream" of owning a home in the suburbs and having a car (or several cars) for free-dom and independence. It was predominantly white middle- and upper-income people who flocked to the suburbs, setting themselves up in well-resourced communities. Housing, land use, and transportation poli-cies reflected this suburban dream—and led to reduced farmland, more high-speed roadways, and less public transit in cities—as well as fewer resources for cities in general.

One result of this shift in population and policy was deteriorating inner cities, which led to and was exacerbated by diminishing tax bases. Even cities that didn't fall into disrepair were deteriorated on other fronts, including having their public transportation systems eroded as people and businesses favored driving. In the San Francisco Bay Area, the pub-lic transportation that preceded today's Bay Area Rapid Transit (BART) system was called the Key System. In the 1940s, a consortium made up of Firestone Tire, Standard Oil, and General Motors—three primary inter-ests invested in advancing the United States' dependence on the car—purchased the Key System under the guise of improving it. Soon thereafter the consortium cited withering revenues as evidence that a more modern system was needed, then proceeded to remove the streetcar tracks and, in many cases, limit bus routes. By ensuring that the system wouldn't function well, the consortium garnered support for its argument that the gutted system was fundamentally flawed. They then set about largely dis-mantling it. Ultimately all three members of the consortium were fined for collusion, but similar "fixes" took place in Los Angeles, Detroit, and other cities as well.

As widespread automobile access increased people's mobility, it spurred a sedentary culture and long commutes that diminished health and increased stress, promoting depression, anxiety, as well as higher rates of chronic diseases.[22] For people who live near major roads and highways, the health impacts of our car-driven culture are particularly acute, includ-ing asthma, heart disease, cancer, and injuries.[23] If we commute an hour a day to and from work, that's seven weeks a year we're spending in a car. If that hour is in traffic, that time comes with stress, poor air quality, and increased risk of a crash.

As suburban sprawl expanded, populating formerly open spaces with housing developments, malls, and traffic, some people became dis-satisfied with the lifestyle. The writer Henry Miller described his dissat-isfaction with the era in his 1945 book *The Air-Conditioned Nightmare*. Although Miller was noted for his then-scandalous books on sex, he found the direction of US changes far more obscene. I remember reading his description of Paradise Point, Long Island, while sitting at that very same beach promontory, one of the primal, still unspoiled parts of the island. By contrast, the countryside and farmland on the parts of the island that sat closer to New York City had transformed into bedroom communities, stretching natural resources such as water supplies and community resources such as school buildings.

SMART GROWTH

The United States continued on its sprawl-centric growth trajectory for most of the twentieth century. In the 1990s, a group of planners, architects, and government administrators organized to create an alternative to development sprawl, a venture they called Smart Growth. Aiming to reduce environmental impact, preserve natural resources, and foster health and safety, the leaders realized Smart Growth could better meet emerging needs.

The Smart Growth approach encourages thinking about the community as a whole and looking at how all the elements in its social and physical composition form an integrated experience that affects health and safety. Smart Growth emphasizes efficient neighborhood designs: housing is typically located within walking distance of shops, services, workplaces, schools, healthy food outlets, as well as a variety of transit and mobility options. The goal is to create functional, accessible, and attractive neighborhoods that are centrally located and have a strong sense of place. Many communities have gone even further, adding health elements to their general or comprehensive plans, as a strategic tool that codifies health in future building decisions.[24] Decision-making ideally engages all constituents, addressing multiple needs and points of view.

Smart Growth first flourished in newer, wealthier, mostly suburban areas that had the financial resources and political capital to achieve results. For many, it promised to alleviate the need for perpetual driving, which is built into suburban life. Many of the first initiatives focused on slow growth, limiting the space and size of new developments, thereby preserving quality of life and limiting environmental impacts.

It wasn't all good. In some cases, Smart Growth was used to control who moved into town—a new form of Not in My Back Yard (NIMBY), which refers to communities of privilege resisting unwanted developments near them. It also forced new potential residents, often those with less money, to move farther out into the exurbs, ironically expanding the takeover of farmland and open space at first, rather than enhancing overall development.

As the Smart Growth movement has grown, it has focused more on innovative, cost-effective ways of fixing what has already taken shape. Increasingly, Main Streets are being restored in small towns, and buildings are being converted for multiple uses in urban areas. This latter trend has drawn many affluent people back to urban settings, where they find more dynamic living—safer streets, wider cultural input, new types of eateries, and a more diverse, creative mix of people. However, renewal carries the risk of disinvested inner cities becoming gentrified, pushing the relatively lower-income residents out altogether. This is, at times, the ironic underside of Smart Growth: the needs of all community members are not always carefully anticipated, and the interests of low-income and non-white communities are—uncaringly—not prioritized. Smart Growth success, for all its practical merits, can and frequently does limit opportunities for the people already living in a neighborhood. As psychiatrist Mindy Thompson Fullilove argues, "In order to design an equitable city, we need to face that there are processes undermining this that have a long history. We must know this history. These processes are constantly evolving."[25]

IMPROVEMENT WITHOUT DISPLACEMENT

For all their virtues, so-called smart changes to existing structures and communities—features that support health such as walking trails, bike paths, healthy food stores, parks, and open space—are often perceived negatively by existing residents and small business owners. They are the first inroads of gentrification, and as they contribute to property-value and demographic changes, they can ultimately lead to displacement of the current residents and businesses—the people the additions should benefit ost. Low-income and particularly Black and Latino residents have ically experienced government and business processes that have diminished their communities or, at a minimum, failed to treat them equal to wealthier white communities; they have to wonder when suddenly their communities advancing.

Dr. Fullilove has described how federal policies, programs, and practices either explicitly or inadvertently displaced generations of families, mostly people of color, repeatedly over history. Examples include segregation, redlining, urban renewal, and the US foreclosure crisis of the early twenty-first century. This serial displacement—forced, recurrent displacement of low-income people of color over time—has profound impacts on community health.[26] First, it disrupts the strong social ties and support networks that long-time neighborhood residents have developed within their communities. Second, when these social connections are broken, this "social loss" creates excess stress and psychological effects, which in turn amplify adverse effects on physical systems that are necessary for resilience against disease and chronic conditions.[27] Dr. Fullilove coined the consequences of this displacement root shock, "the traumatic stress reaction to the loss of some or all of one's emotional ecosystem." Families forced to start over—again and again—lose these vital and intangible resources and in many cases become more susceptible to developing chronic disease. People who have been serially displaced face increased levels of violence in communities, family disintegration, substance abuse, sexually transmitted diseases, and high levels of stress.[28]

The US return to urban areas is, undeniably, pushing lower-income residents out of their neighborhoods. Gentrification is a serious challenge and will remain so as long as there is a shortage of housing and market forces are the only determinant of what housing and commercial property is available and at what price. Some policies that diminish the risks of people being pushed out of their neighborhoods are in place, most notably rent-control protection, but stronger determination and further strategies are needed.

Gentrification often casts low-income populations into the "first ring" of suburbs, those located just outside city limits and where high-polluting industries are often relocated. These areas sometimes have even less infrastructure—such as public transit systems—and less of a tax base than inner cities. They also can have a less organized government structure, making change more difficult. This is why, when improvements to inner-city areas are undertaken, measures should be in place to protect current residents and businesses, such as enforced rent control for individuals and small businesses.

Today, advocates for sustainable development that benefits—rather than displaces—low-income communities of color represent a diverse array of sectors and perspectives. One of them is Oakland architect Mike Pyatok, whose work is internationally renowned for strengthening under-resourced communities through comfortable, practical, and affordable housing that's close to transit.

Pyatok was a central force in a community campaign to include affordable housing in Oakland's Uptown Redevelopment Project, which restored structures such as the Paramount and Fox Theaters to their former grandeur. Pyatok united social workers, developers, homeless people, and faith leaders in a coalition that secured $4 million to build Fox Courts.[29] Both socially and architecturally innovative, this mixed-use, arts-enriched complex near public transportation has won several awards for environmental sustainability. It includes 80 affordable apartments—some reserved for people with HIV/AIDS and others for people with mental illnesses. Fox Courts also provides resources and services such as computer access, employment search assistance, and a homework club for its 125 young residents.

Pyatok's work is part of a broadening movement emphasizing that healthier home design principles should be applied to everyone—not just the privileged. For example, in southwest Minnesota, an affordable 60-unit apartment complex with primarily low-income, ethnically diverse families recently underwent a green renovation. The National Center for Healthy Housing has tracked the effect of this project's green-building principles against health outcomes. Early research shows a majority of adults and children report better health and safety just one year after renovation.[30] The adults improved in areas of general health, chronic bronchitis, hay fever, sinusitis, hypertension, and asthma, while the children benefited in overall health, especially respiratory allergies and ear infections.

LA PLAGE: A ROADWAY TO THE BEACH

I was walking along the street above the Seine River, enjoying a beautiful Paris view on a hot summer night, when I heard Latin music below—a loud, compelling, thumping beat. Finding a ramp, I hurried down to the Seine to join in. Three dancers on a stage led a crowd of at least a hundred in a free Zumba dance session. I was soon sweating and laughing, feeling creative from the sudden and unexpected scene. I might not have been dancing if it hadn't been Paris, where I knew no one.

It turned out the Zumba class was part of what Parisians call La Plage—a section of Paris transformed into a symbolic beach for the summer. As a centerpiece of the theme, a swimming pool had been installed nearby and deck chairs were spread out along the Seine, with people sitting as though they were at the beach. There were beach balls to play with and a water station offering free municipal water Seine-side. A vendor delivered crepes and margaritas to the people lounging on deck chairs. Later I realized this spot was usually the highway, where people commuted to and from town. To get to La Plage, I had taken what was usually the off-ramp of the roadway.

What an amazing community decision—emphasizing health, well-being, surprise, art, and music. Parisians with means often flee the city in the heat of August, but for those who can't, this is a community alternative. When this road was a highway, it was unimaginable that it could be anything else—but now, transformed, it was inconceivable that it could be a highway! I have to credit the vision, courage, and creativity of Parisians and their government. They could look at a roadway and see a dance class, a swimming pool, and a beach.

Efforts like this—in short, turning one's built environment on its head—are seen in the United States as well. Every year, the Philadelphia International Festival of the Arts shuts down Broad Street, the city's major artery leading from its sports stadiums to city hall. Officials roll out sod, laying it over the asphalt, and residents enjoy a wild, free festival filled with music, art, dance, and kids' activities. Up the road, a popup park near the art museum transforms 8 acres of asphalt into a public space filled with giant games of chess and checkers, free music and outdoor movies, and food vendors all summer long. In both cases, it's a lovely exercise in reimagining a gritty, car-dominated space into a hub of community creativity, recreation, and bonding—a reminder of what's possible by changing one's perspective.

TRAFFIC CALMING

Sometimes I begin my prevention presentations with a photo of a traffic-jammed freeway. The mere thought of being stuck in traffic can raise people's blood pressure, which leads me to the first question in my presentation: What are the health issues that come to mind with crowded highways? Most people say stress, then road rage and asthma—all true. Roads' impacts don't end there. Built mostly to accommodate cars, roads and highways discourage other forms of transit—walking, cycling, public transit—in part by not making accommodations for them. As communities make the connection between the design of their infrastructure and the incidence of chronic diseases, health advocates would like to see more people walking and bicycling, safely, to keep their vitality up and their weight down. Constructing sidewalks and safe bike paths is an important aspect of this, as well as ensuring they are designed to be fully inclusive and accessible by all users, including those in wheelchairs. It's the notion of "completing the streets" to meet the needs of all types of mobility. Complete streets make economic sense too: building bike paths produces twice as many jobs per dollar as building roads does.[31] More physical activity also helps reduce the strain on medical and mental health systems.

The notion of "traffic calming" is the designing of roads so the experience of driving on them slows people down—physically and mentally—making it safer and more pleasurable for both motorized and nonmotorized travelers. The strategy aims to complete the streets in a way that merges the social and physical environments, thereby calming both the traffic and the individuals using the roads. A road may curve or narrow from two lanes to one, or it might have protected lanes for cyclists and pedestrians. Mark Fenton, the walking expert, is a big fan of a design technique he calls "bulb-outs," in which sidewalks "bulb" outward at intersections to improve visibility and shorten the crossing distance at street corners. Bulb-outs can also be landscaped and offer seating, adding ambiance and comfort to the street experience.

While traffic calming offers valuable strategies for slowing down cars and trucks, advancing alternatives to these vehicles remains the most important intervention for mitigating the health footprint of our car-catering infrastructure. This isn't easy: a given locality's biggest stream of transportation revenue (or any federal revenue) is the federal transportation bill. Needless to say, it is subject to much vehicle-related lobbying and politics from car-related industries.[32] The auto industry's war on biking has lobbied and marketed to imply that alternatives to driving are humiliating or dangerous. General Motors produced a set of ads for college magazines, one of which depicted a biker who was embarrassed to be seen by peers driving in a car. Another showed a bus whose destination sign read, "creeps and weirdos."[33]

The public can use its influence to advocate for community infrastructure that supports walking, bicycling, and public transit, thus making ads like GM's even more ridiculous. During the reinforcement of the Oakland Bay Bridge during the early twenty-first century, officials said they'd spend whatever it takes to fortify it against earthquakes. Yet, when activists pushed for a pedestrian and bicycle lane, these same politicians claimed the bridge's district couldn't afford it. After an outpouring of public pressure from bicycling coalitions and others, it turned out they *could* afford it after all.[34]

When I-405, a major California freeway, was closed for repairs in 2011, the city of Los Angeles urged everyone to stay home for the weekend. JetBlue took advantage of the news, offering $4 flights to fly the 30-some miles between Burbank and Long Beach airports.[35] As published in *Slate* magazine, "In the face of this fanciful idea . . . it became possible to demonstrate that cycling . . . [was] not only the cheapest form of transportation, not merely the one with the smallest carbon footprint, not only the one most beneficial to the health of its user, but the fastest. A local cycling group, Wolfpack Hustle, bet it could beat the plane . . . [as] others took on the challenge. And guess what? Everyone beat the plane. (Bike: 1:34, Metro/Walk: 1:44, Rollerblades: 2:40, but the plane—with the cabdriver lost on the way to the airport—nearly three hours.)"

Wolfpack Hustle put it this way: "The ride was beautiful and scenic; our race inspired people to roller-skate, to take trains, to walk to the finish.

Meanwhile our politicians and police cowered and bit their nails, telling people to stay home and avoid this sunny California weekend."[36]

Across the United States, more and more communities are realizing the virtues of alternate transportation. Chicago's Active Transportation Alliance is working on complete-streets policies, local bikeways, safe routes to school, and public rallies for safe biking.[37] Atlanta's Pedestrians Educating Drivers on Safety has won policy victories and manages an innovative online system in which residents report barriers to safe walking directly to the appropriate civic agency.[38] Boston's Fenway Alliance, a powerful coalition of 20 well-respected arts, culture, and academic institutions, has improved walkability in Black and Latino districts, revitalizing rich cultural areas.[39] The Wray Health Initiative coalition in rural Colorado has created community buy-in and support for physical activity, as it builds a neighborhood walking path, basketball court, and other facilities.[40]

As Enrique Peñalosa, former mayor of Bogotá, Colombia, puts it, "What really makes the difference between advanced and backwards cities is not highways or subways, but quality sidewalks. . . . An advanced city is not one where even the poor use cars, but one where even the rich use public transport . . . buses and bikeways are democracy in action." He accomplished this in Bogota, adding 2,200 miles of bikeways during his years in office.[41]

THE CASE FOR MY DOG (AND YOURS)

Most mornings I walk my dog, Faroah, at Point Isabel, a shoreline green space and dog park along the San Francisco Bay. Formerly a World War II munitions dump, Point Isabel has been transformed into one of the largest, best dog parks I've ever seen. It's also extraordinarily representative of the diversity of the entire region in terms of race, age, and gender. As is the case in most dog parks, everyone stands around conversing about their dogs, and the atmosphere is light and fun. Without community foresight, this park would have remained a dump. Without Faroah, I would walk a lot less and rarely enjoy the Bay, where I like to contemplate the view and watch the herons, egrets, and other shore birds. As I walk, I see the San Francisco skyline and the Golden Gate and Bay bridges. Having a dog is good for me because of the pleasure of the companionship and the stimulus to stay active.

Although pets provide ample health benefits, environments are built to keep them separate from everyday life, especially in cities. Unlike other countries, the United States keeps dogs out of restaurants, schools, and most workplaces, obsessing over cleanliness and fearing liability. Certainly, some dogs without supervision are a problem. However, US policies imply most pets are problematic or irrelevant, at best, despite extensive research showing their overall value to humans' physical and mental health.[42]

Being with pets counteracts stress and lowers blood pressure, and walking them adds to that effect. Rather than pet dander causing allergies in children, pets help build their immune systems, if the children are exposed from a young age.[43] Dogs can also help children do better at school by improving their focus, and companionship with animals helps kids develop empathy.[44,45] Older people feel less lonely and depressed with pets, and some progressive medical and mental health facilities use pets to lower patient anxiety.[46,47] Animals can also help people in prison by making the environment less intolerable and by reducing fighting, depression, and suicide.[48,49] Animal training programs provide inmates with marketable skills, while helping them build self-esteem, patience, and perseverance, all of which enhance the likelihood of success upon leaving.[50]

Pets humanize cities and towns. I'm lucky to work in a dog-friendly office, where PI deliberately decided that including dogs would lift spirits and personalize the environment. I also see more shop owners with water bowls outside and signs saying, "Dogs welcome," because they realize it's good for business. My favorite restaurant bakes cookies for the dogs, so I'm more likely to eat there, sitting at a heated outdoor table with Faroah at my feet. Pets are also conversation starters and enhance the ambiance of neighborhoods, creating more community vitality.

ARTS AS SOCIAL JUSTICE

Across from Point Isabel, downtown Richmond has experienced ongoing disinvestment since its World War II heyday. But today this area is also home to East Bay Center for the Performing Arts, an example of how a single element of the built environment can have an enormous impact on a community.

The Center is a world-class artistic, cultural, and civic hub that has trained more than 50,000 student artist-leaders. Its vision, shaped by its founder and artistic director Jordan Simmons, is that art can spur social change and that quality arts education belongs to everyone. Adults practice and perform at the Center along with children, making the point that art is a way of life, a way of thinking, and not just an after-school "enhancement."

The renovated Beaux Art building that houses the Center has added to the neighborhood's vibrant revival, enhancing the city in a way that fights gentrification by emphasizing multicultural respect and inclusion. "The idea was that there are beautiful things going on here, so let's make this all glass and allow you to see the dancers, the theater, the movement," architect Mark Cavagnero says. "Let the kids be the life of the building. We want this to have a grittiness and honesty."

This one renovation has had many ripple effects: elevating neighborhood stature and safety, promoting economic growth, and furthering social justice through art and culture. The wave of the future is to create communities where every building block of the built environment—and the way these elements come together as a whole—promotes health in this way.

[5]

THE BURDEN OF UNFAIRNESS

ZIP CODES

I tried to get a mortgage for a superb house in East Oakland near my office, but my application was denied without explanation. Later I learned—off the record—that banks were unwilling to lend in that area. They had "redlined" it, meaning they drew an actual red line on the map around certain neighborhoods where they refused to support either residential or commercial development. This neighborhood was extraordinarily racially, ethnically, and economically diverse, with a high percentage of people of color and people with low household income—typical redlining targets. Wealthier white neighborhoods were, needless to say, not subject to this treatment. Eventually, I was able to get the loan, but only because I had a realtor with a long-standing relationship at the local bank and other business connections that helped me get around the standard practice. Surely the fact that I was a white man with a good income made a big difference—both in my ability to get a realtor and in the bank's willingness to lend money to me. While I had the means and access to buck the system that oppressed others in the neighborhood, the vast majority of East Oakland residents did not.

Redlining and discriminatory lending practices are, of course, not limited to East Oakland—they are part of a much larger pattern of injustice that relegates low-income communities and communities of color to poor health and other forms of diminished well-being. Redlining also reinforces racial and economic segregation while concentrating poverty, poor housing conditions, and overcrowding into set areas,[1] forcing people to live in inequitable conditions that engender poor health. The sum of this is that financial institutions, by restricting housing options, reinforce certain populations to areas with the fewest resources and access to services, jobs, and transportation.[2] This means homes near toxic sites and polluting industries. It's no accident that the leading causes of death—heart disease, cancer, diabetes, stroke, injury, and violence—occur with greater frequency and severity in these areas, and with earlier onset. Further, being denied a path to home ownership becomes a huge barrier to building wealth that can be passed on to the next generation. There is seemingly no end to the unfairness wrought by redlining.

Dr. Tony Iton, Public Health Director of Alameda County (California) from 2003 to 2009 (and also a former board member at Prevention Institute), led a study that found a Black child born in low-income West Oakland and a white child born 10 miles away in the middle-class Oakland Hills had an average fifteen-year difference in life expectancy.[3] As appalling as this finding is, it's only part of the story: life expectancy is a relatively blunt measure that reveals just one element of inequity; it only hints at the lifetime of disparity that accompanies what are too often sicker, shorter lives.

Virtually every US inner city has these kinds of inequities—as do some suburbs,[4] especially those just outside city limits, and many rural areas. Sir Michael Marmot, an international authority on disparities in health, noted in an interview with the World Health Organization: "If you catch the metro train in downtown Washington, D.C., to the suburbs in Maryland, life expectancy is fifty-seven years at the beginning of the journey. At the end of the journey, it is seventy-seven years. This means that there is a twenty-year difference in life expectancy in the nation's capital, between the poor and predominantly Black people who live downtown and the richer and predominantly non-Black people who live in the suburbs."[5]

Sadly, I haven't seen any discernable embarrassment or political fallout over this inequality—or any significant activity to address it in, of all places, our nation's capital. Marmot has revealed the pattern of diverging life expectancy and income levels in countries around the world. In other countries, the discrepancies in life expectancy track economic status. In the United States, racism and economic injustice are deeply intertwined, exacerbating the inequities. The dismaying links between neighborhood conditions and health have been recognized by groups in Washington, D.C., and New York City through the creation of transit maps that show the average life expectancy for residents living around each metro stop. In New York, visual artist and programmer Brian Foo has even used musical narration to map the profound income gaps along a subway line.[6] Public and private projects that are disruptive to neighborhoods, such as electricity substations, freeways, and waste treatment plants, tend to be placed in the very same neighborhoods that are redlined. "This is typical of the pattern you see in poor neighborhoods," according to Meena Palaniappan, an Oakland resident whose concern led to her becoming co-director of the West Oakland Environmental Indicators Project. "Facilities that serve the whole Bay Area are located here, and West Oakland shoulders the whole environmental burden."[7] West Oakland residents suffer from predictably higher rates of lead poisoning, cancer, and asthma. One study shows that local children are seven times more likely to be hospitalized for asthma than the average child in California.

Since the health problems created by inequitable community conditions all eventually require medical treatment and people living with chronic health problems often end up hospitalized, the search for solutions to these disparities in health typically begins in the medical system. The Institute of Medicine has identified three vital elements for achieving greater medical equity: equal access to high-quality treatment, diverse medical leadership that represents the populations served, and treatment that is culturally and linguistically appropriate.

Where this line of thinking goes wrong is in assuming the medical system can play the primary role in solving the problem; as discussed already, inequity isn't just medical. It's a piling on of economic, environmental, and political unfairness. The gap in life expectancy isn't principally due to differences in treatment, or in biological makeup. It's related to ordinary community issues with ignored health impacts that degenerate into medical concerns. As Brian Smedley, the executive director of the National Collaborative for Health Equity, puts it, "It's not your genetic code; it's your zip code."[8] The environments in which people live, work, and play shape health and safety outcomes for everyone—but this impact is *even more so* for low-income populations and people of color, who bear the brunt of injustice manifested in challenging living conditions and social stigmas. As Marmot writes, "It is about opportunities in life . . . social conditions that shape the physical environment one lives in."

THE BOND IS BROKEN

Daisy, a young Latina in Santa Ana, a low-income community in otherwise wealthy Orange County, California, photographed a vacant, fenced-in lot for a creative project called PhotoVoice. She explained her picture this way: "We could use this as a place to play sports. We don't get to interact as much because we don't have places to play. The bond is broken. We could build a park so that kids my age can stay active, healthy, and connected."

A positive environment matters. Nurturing health and well-being is about both the physical conditions of neighborhoods—such as the existence of a park or produce market—and a sense of caring relationships, as Daisy observed. Day-to-day diminishments and degradations are wearing, especially when it's obvious that people in other communities fare much better. ~~People's visceral responses to their surroundings literally shape their sense of self-worth and ability.~~

"I visited my brother in jail this weekend," an Oakland student told Vice President Joe Biden, who was addressing a youth rally. "The jail was cleaner and painted better than my school. What are you saying about me and Oakland when I see that?"

The Oakland school's appearance and the vacant, fenced-in lot in Santa Ana are both literal and symbolic statements, which both youth seemed to perceive and correctly interpret as cues in their environments. Other neighborhoods have well-resourced schools and attractive parks. In the face of these and other inequities, it takes a lot of resilience for Daisy and the Oakland youth to *not* feel less valued by society.

The links between a person's surroundings and his or her feelings of well-being have been studied in matters as simple as trees. At a public housing complex in Chicago, a study compared the experiences of residents who were randomly assigned to apartments that looked out on either trees or a concrete courtyard. Residents living in the units that faced trees reported better neighborhood social ties and community cohesion[9] and a greater sense of safety.[10] In addition, residents facing green space reported improved mental health and well-being, which strengthened their resilience for coping with life issues, such as poverty.[11] In Philadelphia, too, planting greenery in vacant lots in the city was associated with fewer gun assaults and less vandalism over the course of a decade; residents also reported exercising more and feeling less stress.[12]

All children and adults need to feel like they are worthwhile and that they have the support and capacity to make their way in the world. When difficulties in physical surroundings mix with difficulties in social interactions, the interplay of these experiences hits hard, especially for those lacking other strong supports. As Jim Garbarino, a psychologist who studies children's well-being puts it, "No one risk factor accounts for much by itself. It is the overwhelming accumulation without compensatory protective factors that puts kids at risk."[13] When these children grow up and become adults who are unfairly denied access to political and financial resources, the accumulation of risk can take a serious toll on health and life expectancy.

ROBERT MOSES: DISCRIMINATION BY DESIGN

Robert Moses was a city planner in New York City who oversaw the city's development boom during the post-Depression twentieth century. Starting out as a road administrator managing New York City's bridges, tunnels, and roads, Moses became known as the "Master Planner" of mid-century New York and the "Godfather of Urban Sprawl."[14] His widespread influence catalyzed similar approaches to urban planning across the country.

Moses pioneered the notion of "public authorities," a form of power rooted almost exclusively in control of a large revenue stream. In Moses's case, this revenue came via the city's bridges and tunnels, for which he asserted that tolls should be allocated exclusively to building and maintaining roads. Through the Triborough Bridge and Tunnel Authority, Moses leveraged a very large budget into alliances with key unions, whose projects he funded. In short order he exercised this combined clout to build networks of roads, parks, and beaches.[15] Any mayor who challenged him did so at political peril—or, more precisely, political doom.

Moses was a brilliant strategist, but he used his political maneuvering to harm communities of color. His public works projects—parks, pools, playgrounds, beaches—mainly enhanced wealthy, white neighborhoods, many at the expense of poorer areas. An example was Jones Beach, built from a swampy series of several small islands about 20 miles outside city limits. The beach would become a pristine playground for *some* New York City residents, but the road to the beach passed through towns on nearby Long Island. Long Island's officials rejected the building of the roads, prompting Moses to find a loophole.

By calling the road he wanted to build through Long Island a *parkway*, he was able to use small strips of land that New York City already held rights to for piping in water from the Adirondacks. Moses designed these parkways for "restricted travel," as he put it, with low bridges and overpasses, so cars could use them but buses could not. This decision wasn't just anti-Public transit; it was deliberately meant to exclude Black residents who relied on public transit to travel. Once these parkways were built, they ultimately and predictably laid out an infrastructure for upscale suburbs that were accessible only from exits off the parkways. As such, the initial anti-Public transit design for the beach led to more segregation and discrimination, spreading these isolationist "values" to the suburbs.

At the same time, Moses intentionally routed his New York City expressways, which he categorized as being "open to mixed traffic," through the heart of working-class poor areas, like the South Bronx, thereby contributing to the deterioration of the physical integrity, social fabric, and opportunity base of these entire neighborhoods. Thousands of people were displaced with little concern about where they would end up. Referring to these dynamic neighborhoods as "slums," Moses disdainfully boasted to the *Atlantic,*

> It is a curious fact that . . . more slum clearance has been accomplished indirectly than directly—that is, through clearance not for public, semi-public, or private housing, but for parks, playgrounds, parkways, expressways, boulevards, and other public improvements. . . . My particular little group of demolition and building demons have without fanfare and social worker abracadabra pulled down more old rookeries than all the housing experts and

authorities put together. And the best thing about it is that we have substituted nothing for the rookeries but broad highways lined with landscaping and recreation facilities, open to the sun and the elements, and affording the very best incentive to further slum clearance and improvement on their boundaries.[16]

The fact is that after his "public improvements" took full effect, they not only reduced the amount of housing but also helped produce the very slums he claimed to be clearing. Divided by the new highways and literally "in their shadow," the primarily Black and Puerto Rican communities living in the South Bronx's remaining buildings from the 1960s onward had less access to quality jobs, education, and fresh food. The expressway inflicted pollution, noise, and blight, leaving a trail of health and safety problems. Bank redlining of the entire South Bronx made any potential neighborhood improvements impossible despite many residents' commitment to the community. The area's physical degradation was most visible, but the ensuing frustration and hopelessness were perhaps even more devastating.

It has taken decades for resilient residents in the South Bronx to start rebuilding social, economic, and environmental infrastructure. But even as neighborhoods in the South Bronx have begun to improve, many other city neighborhoods have experienced similar dismantling. The prototype Moses established for "urban renewal" has served as the playbook for cities across the country, where new, visually appealing streetscapes, shopping districts, and restricted residential areas help advance prosperity for the wealthy, while dislocating others and destroying the culture and social dynamics of poor, mostly Black and Brown communities. Using vernacular common for the time, New York writer James Baldwin mocked urban renewal efforts as "Negro removal," or racism through infrastructure.

COMMUNITY DETERMINANTS OF HEALTH

When I moved to the culturally rich and economically diverse East Oakland neighborhood, there was a mix of homeowners and renters living in a blend of large apartment buildings and hundred-year-old Victorian and Queen Anne–style houses, some of the most impressive architecture in the city. The residents took pride in their houses, gardens, and the neighborhood, and they were very welcoming to newcomers like me. Some of these homes had deteriorated, but, increasingly, residents were restoring them, often with their own labor. Families with young children visited each other's houses on a regular basis. Though the neighborhood was such a pleasure to live in, redlining reduced investment in and increased violence in the community, which contributed to the fact that it was slower to become gentrified even as wealthier people moved into Oakland.

Decades earlier, when this part of East Oakland was primarily a white neighborhood,[17] disreputable realtors had gone door-to-door attempting to cultivate ire—and new home listings—after the first homes in the area were sold to Black families. The realtors warned of a looming influx of Black people, propaganda meant to generate sales from racist panic, which would in turn allow the realtors to quickly profit by reselling homes at higher prices. But unlike many neighborhoods throughout the state and country, the homeowners in this Oakland neighborhood didn't take the bait; they were comfortable as the neighborhood became increasingly multiethnic. By the time I moved in, the diversity among my housemates was not seen as unusual.

The neighborhood demonstrated what's called "community cohesion"—positive relationships and trust between people of various backgrounds and experiences. Community cohesion improves the safety of the neighborhood—and the feeling of safety—as people are more likely to respect and protect one another and to offer help when someone is in need.

Community cohesion is also an example of what the Prevention Institute calls a *community determinant of health*. It's an idea that came about in the early days of the organization and one that aims to help people put a name to the underlying community issues that foster inequities in health.

To identify these community determinants of health, we reviewed the health literature to identify the aspects of communities that are linked to the top causes of illness, injury, and death. We also looked at the behaviors ost linked to diseases and injuries—such as unsafe driving, vio- ealthy eating, and lack of physical activity. Then we noted ties hese behaviors and neighborhood conditions. So, for example, unhealthy eating was tied to the kinds of foods sold. Road and sidewalk conditions were tied to traffic injuries. The amount of public recreation space was tied to physical activity.

The following is an example of how these ties play out and create inequities between communities. When I lived in East Oakland, I noticed the fresh fruits and vegetables in the supermarkets actually cost more than in the wealthier Montclair neighborhood of Oakland—and the quality of the produce was worse, too. So, not only was it simply more difficult to find healthy food in a poor neighborhood—because big supermarkets avoided doing business there—but healthy food cost more and wasn't as tasty as in a richer area. There was a lack of opportunity in terms of eating healthfully in the poorer area, and this affected behavior.

Once we researched these kinds of inequities in communities, we created a tool to catalogue them. Communities can use the tool to figure out what they need to do in order to reduce inequity, so residents can thrive. In fact, the name of the tool is THRIVE: the Tool for Health and Resilience in Vulnerable Environments.

We categorized the THRIVE factors under three clusters: "people," "place," and "equitable opportunity." Communities with lots of block parties, park clean-ups, and informal socializing on the street are healthier in the "people" sense, as are those that have higher voting rates and a peaceful mix of different races, ethnicities, classes, and gender orientations.

The equitable opportunity cluster relates to factors such as how easy it is to get a good education, a home, and a decent-paying job. Areas with public schools that must wait many months to fill vacant teacher spots aren't as healthy as those where teachers compete for jobs. Neighborhoods where it's hard to get a mortgage due to redlining by banks, or to find a job that pays more than minimum wage, also aren't as healthy in this equitable opportunity sense.

The place cluster includes the physical ("built") environment—the types of businesses, how safe the area is, whether there are venues for artistic and cultural expression. Neighborhoods with billboards advertising mostly unhealthy products, or with lots of liquor stores but few supermarkets, are less healthy in the place sense.

Another place factor—sidewalks—can signal racial inequities that affect health and safety. For instance, the safest and most continuous

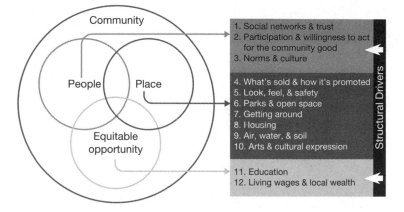

Figure 3   THRIVE Clusters and Factors

sidewalks are often found in neighborhoods that are mostly white and wealthy and where walking is less common. Contrastingly, inadequate or nonexistent sidewalks are most common in Brown and Black neighborhoods, where people are poorer and depend more on walking to get around.[18] To increase health and safety, investments in better sidewalk infrastructure and traffic calming should be prioritized in the neighborhoods where pedestrians are most at risk. By understanding the links between these community determinants, people can work to improve poor conditions—and thus health.

IT STARTED WITH AN INHALER

Thousands of people in West Oakland have worked hard to improve the community determinants of health in their neighborhood, a part of town that was once synonymous with systemic racism, withering economic and educational opportunities, and environmental injustice. But what led to such collective action? It's helpful to consider the individual stories and leadership that have made up the larger progress.

Margaret Gordon is an activist in West Oakland. As she tells it, "I got involved because of an inhaler." In 2000 Gordon went to the nursing office of her neighborhood school, where she observed a nurse with a basket full of inhalers. "I asked, 'Why?'" recalls Gordon. "Well, we had a yeast factory—Red Star Yeast."[19] The location of the factory, combined with Oakland's significant industrial truck traffic, had given rise to local air pollution, which in turn led to a proliferation of asthma, particularly among the more susceptible population of children. Hence: inhalers.

Gordon began doing research in her free time, collaborating with neighbors who were affected. Together, they traced the patterns of illness in their neighborhood back to the major toxic sources. "Asthma, heart disease, respiratory disease—later on it can contribute to high blood pressure," Gordon says. "My neighborhood is so impacted in so many ways. Place matters. That's what enticed me to get involved."[20]

Zeroing in on the Red Star Yeast factory, which was allowed to exceed legal emission limits on foul-smelling carcinogens, residents began taking action to oppose the factory.[21] After a while, the effort received a major boost: the city council chose the Red Star Yeast site, adjacent to the BART station, for a proposed $400 million mixed-use transit village with the goal of adding affordable housing and sustainable jobs.[22] If Red Star didn't close, the city would lose out on its investment. As issues of environmental justice, health equity, and economic incentive braided together, the community vision came into focus, and coalitions collaborated even more closely.

"We had to go out beyond our city and bring in the federal EPA, the county public health department, the state's environmental quality office," Gordon says. The cooperative enlisted community agencies, city council members, and attorneys and also sought the counsel of the Pacific Institute for Studies in Development, Environment, and Security to learn how to establish an evidence base, translate the issues to media, and strengthen political support. "We had a couple of victories," Gordon recalls. Youth groups got involved, launching a clean-air festival and confronting regulators at public hearings "We have an air-monitoring team and community participatory research; we are not totally dependent on academia to come to our neighborhood,"[23] says Gordon.

These efforts succeeded in closing the yeast factory and capping the environmental toxins that had burdened the community since its opening. The transit/redevelopment project at the Red Star site was adopted, and on the high of their collective victory the community went on to successfully tackle other social-justice issues. Gordon and her neighbors' efforts played a big part in prompting the city to pass an ordinance rerouting trucks away from residential areas and onto main roads in 2005; shortly after that, the mayor appointed Gordon commissioner of the Port of Oakland, where she's been developing air-quality plans for shipping companies ever since. And, as a member of the advisory committee for the EPA's Clean Air Act, Gordon now makes sure the community maintains a strong voice and political representation within the regulatory agency.

Margaret's work in mobilizing the community with the Red Star Yeast project is an excellent example of how local leadership can drive change to stem institutionalized social injustice. Supporting community members as leaders and partners builds trust and a common understanding and language, helps identify the most important local priorities and needs, builds on existing community strengths and values, and enhances buy-in from those who will be most affected by the strategies that are put in place.

ED ROBERTS AND THE MOVEMENT FOR EQUAL RIGHTS FOR PEOPLE WITH DISABILITIES

Community is more than a physical place; it's common ground. This is no truer than for people with physical disabilities, who share a bond with one another based on their everyday experiences of navigating the world and how they are viewed by others.

I met Ed Roberts, the legendary leader of the equal rights movement for people with physical disabilities and for independent living, at the airport. Frankly, I was surprised and awed that he was even getting on an airplane; Roberts contracted polio when he was fourteen, and thereafter he had to come to terms with not being able to play sports as well as not being able to walk again. Polio rendered him quadriplegic; he breathed through the "miracle" of an 800-pound iron lung until, against all odds, Ed taught himself to breathe without it. Accompanied that day by his attendant and a daunting array of medical equipment and other supplies, Roberts was pushing it to new limits on cross-country flights to advocate more broadly for the rights of people with disabilities.

Roberts, who died in 1995, was a perceptive, brilliant, and creative man who went on to lead the Center for Independent Living at the University of California at Berkeley, the mission of which is to provide services, support, and advocacy to enhance the rights and abilities of people with disabilities. "Most people never thought of independence as a possibility when they thought of us," Roberts once said. And indeed, when Ed had applied to the University of California at Berkeley in the 1960s, one of the deans remarked, "We tried cripples, and that didn't work."

One of Roberts's tactics for dismantling stigma and prejudice was to introduce the concept of universal design (or universal access), which emphasized commonalities among people instead of differences. A remarkable victory for Ed's group was to secure the country's first curb cuts, the sloped ramps that usually lead from the sidewalk to a crosswalk. For a pedestrian on two feet, they might go unnoticed, but for a mother with a stroller or a person with a walker or in a wheelchair, they're a small innovation that eases the transition to the street. When Ed was working on the issue, some legislators disdainfully mocked, "Why do you need curb cuts? We never see people with disabilities out on the street. Who is going to use them?" After the curb cuts were put in place, the community discovered that many others benefited from them as well, such as elderly folks and people pushing strollers or riding bikes. As Roberts explained, "So many people benefit from this accommodation. This is what the concept of universal design is all about."[24]

Later in life, on the first day of his job as director of the California Department of Rehabilitation, Roberts was riding the elevator when he heard two people next to him talking. They obviously hadn't even noticed him; he was used to being overlooked. One of the men said, "Hey, I hear we're getting a new boss. It's a cripple." Roberts looked at them, smiled, and said, "Allow me to introduce myself. I'm Ed Roberts, your new boss."[25]

UNLOCKING THE TRAP OF ASSUMPTIONS

Everyone, everywhere is affected by cultural attitudes and assumptions based on traits such as gender, race, disability, and class. Often these are so deeply embedded that people don't realize they exist. , born with spinal muscular atrophy, talks about this in his *le Boy Grows Up: How the Disability Rights Revolution Saved My* e hidden assumptions about disability that lurk behind seemingly innocuous statements from strangers, such as "It's so beautiful to see you outside today." As Mattlin writes, "Worse still are the remarks directed at whoever is with me that demean us both: The people who ask my African-American friends if they're my nurses. Or ask my wife if I'm her brother—or even, once, her son!—based on an assumption that someone like me wouldn't have friends or a spouse."[26]

Whether conscious or not, stereotypes and prejudices are scarring. In the United States, their impact is heightened by the culture of heroism, which perpetuates a notion that all barriers can be overcome through sheer will. This fosters a culture of blaming individuals (and individuals blaming themselves) in cases where they flounder or fail—*even if* they know that the environment is slanted against them and that prejudice is unjust and *even if* they recognize that other environments are much more privileged than theirs. It is difficult not to internalize lack of opportunity as failure.

The debilitating effect of ongoing prejudice was aptly named "weathering" by Dr. Arline Geronimus, who studies the cumulative impact of racism. Weathering manifests in the body in measurable ways, in particular the release of cortisol, the fight-or-flight hormone, which creates a state of perpetual anxiety. Over time, cortisol and its associated stress compromise the immune system and can erode people's mental health, alter behavior, and lead to other health risks, such as higher smoking rates, poor nutrition, and earlier pregnancies.

Geronimus's work has shown that the weathering effect isn't limited to people with low incomes. Wealthier, successful African Americans, especially women, experience weathering from ongoing exposures to prejudice and discrimination, including racism and sexism. Weathering even gets into the genes: the emerging field of epigenetics has shown how our genetic code can be imprinted with the effects of these sorts of traumas, then show up in the next generation.[27,28] Trauma becomes hard-wired in a family, a community, or an ethnic or racial group, and as ongoing adversities compound, dignity and hope tend to diminish.

Every step we can take to restore dignity and hope is essential. Brian *HR*
Smedley calls this the "opportunity agenda"—that is, a mandate to systematically focus on the community changes that emphasize opportunity,
hope, and options for success for all. I believe that communities more
clearly taking control of their own agendas and advocating against oppres-
sive assumptions is both a strategy and a confirming end in itself. This
dynamic was embodied by the Black Panthers emphasizing Black power
and Black pride, along with lesbian and gay rights movements and many
other grassroots actions and movements.

Involvement in the arts can be a transformational way to increase hope
and opportunity. The Mural Arts Project in Philadelphia,[29] a grassroots
effort that engages community members in the creation of murals citywide, transforming otherwise depressed and blight-filled neighborhoods
into public art displays that cultivate local pride and reflect community
culture, history, and vision.

Through art, people are able to assert their own authentic voice and
vision in the face of systems that chronically undermine their dignity.
I saw the Atlanta Youth Choir perform twice, and they were riveting in
their energy and enthusiasm. Their words struck me as a simultaneous
cry for help ("Everywhere I go there are guns. . . . Can't sleep because the
enemy is around"), a statement of reality ("Guns are our game and guns
are our ball"), and a message of hope ("Another day, another year, a chance
to get it right"). The choir members were using their collective voices to
demand change and to envision a better future.

BOYS DON'T CRY

*I remember my mother telling me at age four that I cried too easily. I was
too sensitive; boys don't cry. I became very embarrassed and had to learn to
hide, even deny, my feelings. Having internalized her messages about male
character—confirmed by the world around us—I still sometimes find myself
acting too confident and too tough, trying to push down what I feel instead of
understanding and confirming it.*

*As I grew up, I learned about displaying the "right" kinds of male attri-
butes: bold, confident, smart, brawny, and dominant. Some kids at school said*

I threw a baseball like a girl. I felt humiliated and tried to figure out how to throw differently. They called me "gay," which until then had seemed like a positive word, an old-fashioned word for happy; this puzzled me. Once I figured out what it meant, their words stung me and made me concerned I might be effeminate, which I was meant to understand was not acceptable. I was supposed to be stronger and cleverer than girls. Anything else would have been diminishing— or, to put it more precisely, emasculating. So I had to be assertive in class and always have the right answer first.

There didn't seem to be any room for questioning the societal expectations of my childhood. I tried to take on the knowledge subtly, as though the ideas were inherent to me. The subtlety by which these messages were delivered—literally "in the air"—made me feel a tremendous pressure and shame from not knowing, let alone from not manifesting, the "right" set of qualities. Fear of humiliation from not getting it right always loomed; I felt like a tourist who didn't know how to behave in a country not my own. Pressures to be "manly" drove me, and still drive men, to succeed at all costs, ignore risks, and resist support. It weakens any sense that we should all get to determine who we are and what we feel.

And it turns out some of these "manly" norms are also bad for health. As an adult, I was introduced to Kate Millett, a pioneer of the term "sexual politics" and author of a book of the same name. By then, I was well aware of the ways that our culture limits and damages us with its strong gender norms, but I still didn't entirely understand what sex, gender, and politics had to do with one another. As Millett wrote, "There remains one ancient and universal scheme for the domination of one birth group by another— the scheme that prevails in the area of sex." Many of Millett's conclusions came from studying racism—how it operates as oppression and the kinds of responses needed to challenge and overcome it.[30]

Millett articulated women's relentless fight for control over their own bodies in relation to safety, reproductive health, and choice. She confronted the stigma of women being less competent and less rational and how this is translated into their being undervalued and underpaid in the workforce. She spoke out against societal taboos and the way women are first victimized and then even blamed and denied help for revealing domestic violence or rape. It takes an insistent outcry for people to see how gender assumptions play out in damaging health effects.

Hearing Millett's arguments helped me put words to what I experienced as a child. She brilliantly articulated how diminishing women's roles, capacity, and power was harmful to them and influenced their experiences, opportunities, health, and safety. I realized how these polarizing norms limited men as well—both men who were comfortable within the norms and those who questioned them. These expectations lead to some men feeling inadequate if they aren't risk takers or career successes. Expectations of toughness can lead to risky behavior and a cavalier attitude toward preserving one's health. As men's health expert Will Courtenay argues in his book *Dying to Be Men*, "Men's and boys' behaviors and health practices are a major determinant of their excess mortality and premature deaths. . . . One half of all men's deaths each year in the United States could be prevented."[31]

It was a bit controversial at that point for a man to call himself a feminist, but it gave me an important way to express my support and commitment to change. I didn't know then that I would later dedicate part of my work to understanding the influence of norms on behaviors and health. Prevention Institute has helped to define the underlying norms that shape expectations of how men and women "should" act. These norms include equating manhood with aggression, control, and dangerous risk-taking behavior—and too often, victimizing women and children. They include limited roles for women, such that women are encouraged, subtly and overtly, to act and be treated as objects that are used and controlled by others, often men.

At about age eight I learned that I was supposed to be interested in girls. Of course, I was already interested in girls and in boys —we all played together— but now I was becoming aware of distinctions that related to my growing up successfully. Clearly, chasing girls, especially the ones with the most "value" ascribed to them, was part of growing up right. As I aged, the information became more sexual. Still, it didn't make any real sense and didn't particularly conform to the boys and girls I liked, our developing bodies, or my innate judgment.

Over time, my parents devolved from saying that my older cousin Jerry was "like that" to calling him a "fairy." "Fairy" was another word that seemed positive and appealing but certainly not masculine. Jerry didn't have a wife or children, like men were supposed to have. My family treated him warmly and yet as if he were a misfortunate soul—somehow disabled. I had always loved spending time with Jerry at family gatherings. Yet despite his being warm, caring, and creative, I understood that he wasn't supposed to be a role model for me.

Even though my family never said out loud that we should be hostile toward gay and lesbian people, they treated them with disregard. At best, so did much of the rest of society, but often it went much further than that, transforming personal states of affairs into brutal mistreatment and denying people fundamental safety and rights. Around the corner from my house, an empty storefront was made into a French café, but my parents said to stay away. Of course, that made me more curious. It was only open at night, and the café curtains were drawn, yet there was lots of traffic in and out. I looked in during the day and noticed its attractive pillars, with art posters and French café chairs—the kind of look I gravitate toward. I was told "fairies" hung out there. I was told that the crowd was virtually all men, yet peeking through the curtains I noticed many looked more like women. Once in a while, the police would pull up, a massive number of cars with their lights flashing, and they would haul people out and arrest them. I saw the humiliation and fear on many of their faces. "How unfortunate to be that way," I thought, never questioning why they were being arrested and whether it was justified. I understood the world was this way and that I had to navigate carefully to fit into its constraints.

As I got older, I began to understand the stigma and how a sense of "otherness" could make someone feel worthless and ashamed, even if they were being true to who they were. I realized none of the TV shows, magazines, or ads showed people who were anything but heterosexual. The stigma and exclusion were so strong that mainstream culture entirely omitted people who in any way didn't conform to expected sexual orientation or gender identity. Beyond exclusion, gay, bisexual, transgender, queer, and questioning people (LGBTQ) have frequently been treated with violence, discrimination, bullying, and negative stigmatization. Later in life, I started to have a lot of close LGBTQ friends and re-explored my own sexuality and gender. I enjoyed the liberated feeling of being beyond the rules I had grown up with and being part of something unconventional. At the same time, I felt the sting of stigma in a more personal, outraged sense and started to understand the venom lurking behind the stigma. I had friends whose own families abandoned them. Such isolation and pain were unimaginable to me, though so familiar to them.

Understanding how isolation takes a toll on physical and emotional health, it makes sense, sadly, that higher rates of alcoholism, depression, and suicide are observed among those who are treated differently due to their gender or sexual orientation. LGBTQ youth make up about 40 percent of all homeless youth in the United States, primarily because of rejection and/or abuse by their families.[32] They are also significantly overrepresented in the juvenile justice system—which is woefully ill-prepared to serve them—due to exposure to abuse and violence, substance abuse, homelessness, and biased school policies.[33,34]

I spent a lot of my childhood feeling confused by societal expectations of who I was "supposed" to be and who I really was, a dissonance that made me feel shame and doubt where I should have felt self-respect and dignity. I had the advantages of being a white male in a working-class family, but this experience helped me to understand how societal pressures affect everyone who is treated a certain way due to their race, gender, ethnicity, or other monolithic characteristics. It helped me see how a feeling of confusion and powerlessness plays out and is amplified in whole communities that are oppressed simply for their race, sexual orientation, gender, and/or ability, instead of being respected and cherished as individuals.

The United States has seen some real progress toward challenging stereotypes and prejudice in the last decade. The "Don't Ask, Don't Tell" law, which kept LGBTQ people from openly serving in the military, was repealed, and the Supreme Court determined that same-sex marriage is protected and legal in all states. These shifts open the door for norms change and further policy changes that are still needed to address continued inequality and silencing of LGBTQ populations. Workplaces are also implementing greater protections against sexual harassment and expanding parental leave policies. Awareness of sexual assault against women on college campuses and in the military has increased. And in popular culture, women of color are being cast in more dynamic and powerful roles on television and being revered as feminist icons through their music.

Norms are changing, not just in the United States but across the world. When I was in South Africa to speak at a World Health Organization meeting, I visited the Sonke Gender Project, which promotes healthy norms related to men and women. At the time, there was a popular T-shirt being marketed to young girls across the country, which read, "I'm too pretty to study, so my brother does my homework."[35] *This made the Sonke staff angry—why wouldn't a girl believe it's more important to be pretty than intelligent, when the pervasive culture reinforces that notion?* Why wouldn't boys also take for granted that girls should have good looks instead of brains—and certainly not both—and focus their interest on the attractive ones? *So Sonke organized with local communities and picketed some of the box stores selling the shirts, and soon they were off the shelves across the entire country. In the United States, where there were no protests, companies showed no concern, and the shirts remained on the shelves.*

It's a different world for boys and girls than the one I grew up in—and, I think, a more accepting one. Progress has been made and much further progress is needed.

A MOVEMENT FOR EQUITY

It's an exciting time; the national dialogue on gender and race is expanding and the legal rights and opportunities of individuals with mental and physical disabilities are broadening. While there is greater readiness for change in some ways, there is also an urgency to go much further and much faster, an urgency born of frustration with the palpable injustices that persist. Black Lives Matter and Occupy Wall Street[36] are but two recent movements that speak equally to impatience with the slow pace of social justice and civil rights and to the passion and need to accelerate change in institutions and laws at the same time as behaviors and norms.

On a recent trip to Memphis, I visited the Civil Rights Museum, a simple and unpretentious name for the Lorraine Motel, the spot where Dr. Martin Luther King Jr. was shot. I had forgotten he was in Memphis to defend the rights of sanitation workers on a day too stormy to work, when white workers were paid for eight hours and Black laborers were sent home without pay after two hours. It was another typical injustice to be endured as part of the reality of racism—or, as Dr. King rightly saw it, to be challenged. As he reflected, "Laws only declare rights. They do not deliver them." The museum housed the very bus Rosa Parks rode when she refused to move to the rear. On the outside, in large block letters, an advertisement read: "Why fight traffic? Go by bus." Such a contemporary message, probably the same as on some of the buses we ride today, made me realize just how recent some transformations are.

The historic struggle for civil rights in the South conjures an image of Black–white confrontation and growing Black political power. It also brings to mind important Black–white alliances. Experiencing this museum against the backdrop of Memphis, historically a racially divided city that's now multiethnic, I was sure it wasn't accidental that the first display started with an exhibit emphasizing the discrimination that Latinos have faced in this country. Next, it showed a Jewish woman of Polish descent who wasn't allowed to attend school, then a Japanese-American who fought for the United States in World War II while his family was sent to an internment camp.

The museum recognized that different elements of discrimination are related. And therein lies an opportunity: to combine the efforts of communities fighting for equity and justice in order to form a stronger movement overall. Currently communities working on different equity issues share certain values, but much of the practical outreach is moving in parallel instead of being integrated. These strands include the women's movement; LGBTQ, racial, and ethnic empowerment; and physical and mental disability rights. Each has its own compelling issues that could achieve more by deliberately joining together. A collective could become transformative.

Helen Keller saw the common thread in different struggles for justice and the power of linking them to a common cause. Though most widely known for her writing about her disabilities, Keller was also a powerful, inspired activist. As a talented deaf and blind person, she was heralded as a national and international hero. But in addition to championing the rights of deaf and blind people, she also helped to found the American Civil Liberties Union (ACLU) and supported the nascent National Association for the Advancement of Colored People (NAACP) and feminist movement. When she started talking about race, she was publicly ostracized. But she wasn't deterred. "My work for the blind . . . has never occupied a center in my personality," Keller wrote. "My sympathies are with all who struggle for justice."[37]

The founders of the Black Lives Matter movement also clearly see and embody the thread that runs through all fights for equity. Started by three Black queer women, Alicia Garza, Patrisse Cullors, and Opal Tometi, after George Zimmerman failed to be indicted for the murder of Trayvon Martin, Black Lives Matter "is an ideological and political intervention in a world where Black lives are systematically and intentionally targeted for demise. It is an affirmation of Black folks' contributions to this society, our humanity, and our resilience in the face of deadly oppression. We are talking about the ways in which Black lives are deprived of our basic human rights and dignity."[38] It also works to "affirm the lives of Black queer and trans folks, disabled folks, Black-undocumented folks, folks with records, women and all Black lives along the gender spectrum. It centers those that have been marginalized within Black liberation movements. It is a tactic to (re)build the Black liberation movement . . . [and it argues that] when Black people in this country get free, the benefits will be wide reaching and transformative for society as a whole."[39]

Much of the leadership in today's struggle for equity will rightfully come from people experiencing injustices. At the same time, people who may not directly experience injustice as frequently also have a responsibility—and ideally a *self-insistence*—to be responsive to the needs of those directly affected and to exhibit the compassion and action that will lead to community and national change.

Social justice is about individual leadership, but it's more about the leadership of communities. Rosa Parks's insistence on dignity was part of a greater voice at the time that raised awareness, orchestrated strategies, and catalyzed action. The community had reached a tipping point, and the same web of support that helped prepare Parks was also nurturing many other grassroots activists, who would be projected as leaders demanding justice.

Parks trained at the Highlander Center, which was originally established to help white laborers organize during the Depression and then turned to training civil rights leaders in the 1950s. The same tactics for and spirit behind one fight—for trade unions—were used for another: civil rights.

Parks, King, and many others learned the civil rights anthem, "We Shall Overcome,"[40] at Highlander, where it was written as a union song. It became the unofficial anthem of the civil rights movement and, really, a cry for universal justice, with an emphasis on joining together so all may succeed.

[6]

FOOD FOR THOUGHT

PURPLE CAULIFLOWER AND A STICK OF MARGARINE

When I was in graduate school, I was looking for a scenic, quiet place to live. My university was on Long Island, 50 miles east of New York City, and I decided to explore communities that were farther out on the eastern tip. It wasn't the fashionable part, with the Hamptons and Montauk Point, but the North Fork, made up of mostly agricultural communities and small towns. By early in the winter I'd found a wonderful old farmhouse tucked away along a bluff. From there, I could make my way through blackberry thickets and down the 70 steps leading to the beach.

The realtor had been hesitant to even show me the property. Though structurally sound, it obviously hadn't been used in ages. The bathroom still worked, but there was no shower, and during the entire year I was there, the water ran brown from decades of rusting pipes. Exiting the bathtub was like emerging from a tanning salon. It was beyond rustic; I might have called it uninhabitable if it weren't for my imagination and daily access to the breathtaking, endless beach. I wasn't bothered by the fact that it had no refrigerator because I figured it would surely be cold enough most of the year to store things on the windowsill. Sure enough, when I aired out the place, I actually found a stick of margarine on the windowsill. At first glance, I thought it might have dropped off the assembly line recently, but after reading the label, I realized, to my amazement, that it dated back to the beginning of World War II—the last time the house had been occupied.

I had more surprises in the spring. My house was sitting on acres of deep purple—purple cauliflower, which I had never seen before. Long Island was rich in food production in those days, and this land was leased to a local farmer. Small farmers thrived by growing a diversity of foods that have since virtually disappeared from our mainstream food system. Purple cauliflower, a centuries-old heirloom from South Africa, flourished in this nutrient-rich soil and bathed in moist sea air. To my delight, this hardy companion was a healthy food. I would cut it fresh and sauté it whenever I prepared a meal—from farm to table before it came into fashion—in perhaps half an hour. It had a delicious, delicate flavor—and it didn't require margarine.

So I had two extremes at my home—the dream of purple cauliflower and the nightmare of thirty-year-old, still "perfect" margarine. As someone who loves to cook and entertain, I enjoyed watching friends' reactions to these two marvels. The margarine inevitably produced shock and dismay, taking away people's appetites. The cauliflower, on the other hand, had a way of perking up a dish and lifting moods, owing greatly to its vibrant color. The full purple effect started in the fields. Seeing my home tucked in the rolling violet blankets, friends would wonder about its taste and texture as they approached, wanting to know the story behind it, where it came from, how it got here.

Food is an everyday expression of our culture, and every cultural identity is partly tied to a unique way of preparing it. Since our survival requires consumption of food, our culinary traditions have reflected our history, both in terms of the land where our ancestors lived and what that land produced. Human ingenuity and community traditions added these basic materials, still reflecting a local ecosystem and its resources. As food cultures have been passed down through the generations, families and communities inherited their knowledge and rituals, which have had an enduring personal and shared significance.

So how, then, did the modern US food system move toward the bionic margarine? From cultivation and processing to marketing and transportation, modern-day food consumption patterns have been reshaped by corporate food production. In a relatively short time span, with developments in technology, aided by agricultural policies, industry changed its emphasis from the marketing of whole foods to manufacturing highly processed food products. Initial innovations, like frozen fruits and vegetables or tomato sauce, had significant benefits, but the drive for profit has led to much greater and more extensive changes, including reduced standards for what constitutes "food."[1]

Consumers welcomed the food industry's innovations, in part because they lowered prices, reduced risks from spoilage, and extended availability beyond the growing seasons. Meals could be prepared more quickly, so women (in traditional roles) were able to spend less time in the kitchen. Women who worked were expected to continue to prepare meals, so convenience was perhaps even more important. Snappy marketing campaigns capitalized on consumer interest in ease and thrift.

Over time, industry and retailers altered the types of available foods and shifted national eating habits, concocting handy foods that were fun, fast, cheap, and tasty. But behind the alluring novelties and happy marketing is a reductionist science that *breaks down* food into nutrients infused with addictive additives and treats our food like a jigsaw puzzle—with the hubris to assume industry can outdo nature and put all the pieces back together again. Subsidized additives—by-products of corn and soy—have allowed manufacturers to modify "recipes" for greater profit.[2] Instead of nature, health, and culture guiding food decisions, business interests became the driver. These changes have caused a radical shift in norms and a host of food-related health impacts.

Nutrient-dense, whole foods—like fruits, vegetables, grains, nuts, seeds, and legumes—that have sustained people for generations have been replaced by the three additives selected to make us buy and consume more—sugar, salt, and fat. Michael Jacobson, head of the Center for Science in the Public Interest and author of terms like *liquid candy*, coined the term *junk food.* Dr. Wendel Brunner, the public health director I worked for in Contra Costa County, goes even further by calling this food *toxic waste.*

I wasn't surprised when the National Cancer Institute announced recently that nearly 40 percent of the calories US youth consume are empty ones, coming from items like soda, pizza, and desserts.[3] In fact, few US youth eat the recommended amounts of fruits and vegetables.[4] The predictable results of these trends have included epidemics of chronic diseases such as diabetes, heart disease, and stroke, all of which have roots in unhealthy eating and inactivity[5] and have seen their onset occurring increasingly in children and adolescents. In a US healthcare model in which disease is treated rather than prevented, the costs associated with these trends have, of course, been astronomical. As the former chief

Centers for Disease Control and Prevention medical coroner Dr. Beverly Coleman Miller once told me, even the organs of children and adolescents are changing: in examining the bodies of inner-city youth who died early—too often from violence—she was shocked to find that their internal organs were damaged to an extent she had previously only seen with older adults.[6]

WOULD YOU LIKE SODA OR WATER?

Soda epitomizes the modern food system and its ripple effects on health. No one has demonstrated this better than Dr. Dick Jackson of the University of California's Fielding School of Public Health,[7] who conducted a mock "Health Impact Assessment" of sodas. Health impact assessments are usually employed to evaluate the potential community health effects of a project or policy before it is approved; Jackson was being somewhat cheeky, albeit brilliantly so, in employing this model to shed light on alternatives that may be better for health and community. Jackson's model demonstrated soda's vast health and environmental impacts as well as its economic costs. Soda, which originated as an occasional treat at the soda fountains in eras past, grew into a daily drink and is now a multiple-times-a-day drink, achieved through skillful marketing, product formulation, and consumer uptake.

Jackson's assessment began with corn syrup, the inexpensive core ingredient that makes soda sweet and cheap. Agricultural corn production for syrup absorbs massive amounts of tax subsidies and fossil fuels, and in turn the extensive use of growth fertilizer contaminates our water,[8] though any sugar source would be similarly problematic. Aluminum and glass production for the soda packaging increases demand for fuel and adds to greenhouse gases in the earth's atmosphere. Transporting soda over long distances to people who could otherwise be drinking healthy tap water increases oil imports and elevates the demand for and price of gasoline. Soda advertisements and billboards create visual pollution. Soda's consumption inflicts extensive medical costs from its associated maladies— bad teeth from sugar, bad livers from all the fructose, bad gallbladders from all the fat formed from excess calories, bad pancreases and diabetes from the weight gain, and increased rates of asthma, pulmonary diseases, and cancers from its transport. Examining all these medical, dental, and environmental costs, we realize ~~even though soda may seem reasonably priced at the register, it is wildly expensive when we tally up the personal~~ and societal costs.

Recognizing soda's direct effect on children's health, Prevention Institute's statewide coalition for healthy eating and physical activity made water a top platform priority in 2008. Several partner organizations— notably the Central California Regional Obesity Prevention Program and California Food Policy Advocates—helped to elevate it on California Governor Schwarzenegger's agenda. The argument was simple: water is a critical asset, and everyone should have a right to it, particularly those who are frequently denied it in rural and low-income communities. Initial inroads on this cause were flawed, as activists tried to find win-win compromises for reducing soda consumption while also benefitting business—specifically, that manufacturers, many of whom also produce soda, sell water instead. This always struck me as a misguided approach: the human need for water is too great for it to be commoditized and made inaccessible to those short on resources. Devastatingly, in the Central Valley, California's premier growing region, water is frequently contaminated with pesticides from crops and chemicals from fracking, so the very people who help feed the nation are deprived of basic sustenance. The need for safe water is urgent and timeless.

At a small lunch with the governor in advance of a healthy food summit in California, colleagues and I shared a study that found roughly three quarters of California schoolchildren did not have access to free, clean drinking water in food-service areas[9]—something unthinkable in the United States, unthinkable in California. The governor was outraged by our findings and later announced at the summit that he would pass a law to fix the problem. One reporter asked how he'd pay for such a bold move in these difficult economic times. The governor acknowledged the cost in providing every kid with clean drinking water and said he was allowing two to three years to figure it out. I understood this—many states and locales were in a fiscal environment where infrastructure projects could be difficult to finance. At the same time, I think there is a real opportunity to recognize the long-term investment in such projects. Part of reimagining our infrastructure in support of health and sustainability is recapturing the ingenuity that has fueled valuable US projects like the Works Progress Administration. I was glad the governor said, "We will do it, no matter how." In 2010, in his final months in office, Governor Schwarzenegger made good on his commitment by signing Senate Bill 1413—legislation that required all California school districts to provide free drinking water during meals. As the administration changed, health advocates have continued to keep the focus on water; in 2015 Governor Brown signed into law a bill that prioritized the funding for water quality and infrastructure in the state's schools.

FOOD JUSTICE AS CRUSHED GRAPES AND FOOD IN THE BELLY

When I lived in New York, the movement to support farmworkers and their union caught fire. The effort was led by Cesar Chavez, who insisted that farmworkers shouldn't be taken advantage of, regardless of citizenship status. Farmworkers were the purveyors of the nation's rich food supply, and the horrendous conditions in which they worked were overdue for change. Farmworkers have a long history of exploitation and systematic deprivation in the United States, and industrial farms' financial bottom lines have long been in conflict with humane treatment of their workers.

As part of the strategy to support the farmworkers' union, Chavez joined New York activists in organizing a boycott of a common non-union farm product: grapes. As a practical matter, this boycott amounted to a total boycott of all grapes, since agribusiness interests had grown so influential that they precluded any union-benefitting negotiations. The greatest sacrifice came from the grape-picking workers, who made the difficult sacrifice of not working even though they desperately needed the pay; the local boycott effort I participated in and the actions I and others undertook in supermarkets seemed paltry in comparison. Chavez, showing what made him a great organizer, attended boycott meetings to emphasize that our boycott, starting in New York and spreading across the country, was critical. He said it also gave a boost to the farmworkers to see the New York news and know that people there were supporting them.

The boycott extended beyond abstaining from grape purchases. To make the issue more relevant for retailers, boycotters would go to local supermarkets and follow a consistent strategy during busy hours: select non-union grapes from the supermarket produce department, place them at the bottom of the shopping cart, then load heavy canned and bottled food on top of them. At checkout, the register worker would add everything up, with the packaged grapes last. At that moment, we boycotters would ask, "Wait a minute, wait a minute—these grapes don't seem to be union-picked!" The cashier would invariably say, "No, they're not," or "I don't know." Then the managers would come to the register and in turn be told by we the customers, "I just can't buy non-union grapes."

It was a bit of a mess, with lots of mushy grapes filling the counter and frustrated people waiting in line. And as we exited the supermarkets, our laughter was admittedly mixed with a little remorse for the sake of the staff. But the message was sent, and the efforts were in some way appreciated by the cashiers (many of them union members themselves). As the ranks of boycotters and inconvenient register scenes grew in number, more supermarkets agreed to purchase only union grapes. When they discovered that no union grapes were available because grape growers had yet to sign any union contracts, the supermarkets didn't carry grapes at all. The boycott and its associated press attention grew so broad-based that supermarkets posted signs in their windows saying, "We don't sell non-union grapes." Over time, more and more farms reached agreement with the union to employ union workers and promote livable wages.

WHERE'S THE FRUIT?

Food and beverage manufacturers have grown increasingly sophisticated in creating the perfect alchemy of products designed to accommodate heavy doses of sugar, salt, and fat, plus pleasing flavorings, coloring, and even *sound profiles* (chips designed to make the most satisfying crunch possible, or sodas packaged to produce the crispest pop and fizzle of carbonated water). Food and beverage producers spend staggering amounts—on the order of billions of dollars—marketing these foods in the United States. The three Ps—pricing, placement, and promotion—for all types of consumers, including children, ensure that highly processed products make

How could HC use this strategy?.

their way into grocery and convenience stores, carts, and homes for any-one who isn't expressly trying to avoid them.

Advertising tactics show that no child is considered too young to start experiencing brand loyalty, on TV and on the Internet, where tactics like food "adver-games" (branded interactive games aimed at specific users) enable marketers to engage children for unlimited lengths of time to promote primarily unhealthy foods.[10] Saturday cartoons run one food commercial for every five minutes of broadcasting, most of them for products that would be objectively labeled junk food. A 2007 University of California at Los Angeles study[11] showed the ads' appeal increases the likelihood children will try those foods and continue eating them, increasing risk for weight gain. Powerful product placement, where the marketing is a part of the story, makes the ads even more tangible.

Marketing companies are employed to sell products at any cost, and as consumers we have allowed them to trade values of health and moderation for our ease of cheap consumption and their profit motives. But even amid recent progress, to stem the tide of unhealthy product marketing, corporations and marketing schemes have managed to co-opt ideas like health and moderation. In cases where it's clear people care about health, especially parents, marketers sell fictional health where it doesn't exist.

The tension between consumers' desire for healthy products and producers' desire to sell cheaper products that are decidedly *unhealthy* is waged on food labels. In 2007, the Prevention Institute conducted a study called "Where's the Fruit?"[12] We examined the products with packaging that used images and wording to imply that fruit would be found in their ingredients, and the results revealed how hard it is to make the healthy choice.

Examining hundreds of the foods most advertised to kids came with some initial good news: manufacturers and marketers were clear that references to fruit are an effective strategy to reach parents and children. In fact, 39 of the 100 foods examined displayed fruit on their packages, either in large letters or, more often, as an attractive illustration. Where the marketers didn't care nearly as much was in the truthfulness of this advertising. Almost half of the 39 products had no fruit whatsoever in the actual product, and most of the rest had very little. Even the few products with more than a tiny bit of fruit almost always had more sugar than fruit.

Just as subversive were front-of-package labels—symbols on the products that suggest nutrient levels or ingredients not actually contained in the products. People have grown to trust these labels since the American Heart Association first introduced its "heart healthy" packaging symbol in 1995—placing a picture of a heart on food labels as a visual marker for healthier options. Picking up on this cue, food manufacturers co-opted front-of-package labeling. Using their own self-developed criteria for nutritional value, they designated a list of products they claim are nutritious enough to be advertised as healthy foods to consumers under the age of twelve. The industry characterizes these products as "better for you"; "less worse" would be more accurate. The Prevention Institute examined the nutritional profiles of fifty-eight products with these front-of-package labels, part of a study called "Claiming Health," because staff discovered that over four out of five of those products failed to meet one or more nutrient criteria. Over half of the overall products and 90 percent of the snack foods analyzed were high in sugar; nearly a quarter were high in saturated fats[13]—a brazen case of false health claims.

In a culture of deceptive marketing, it's clear more should be done to protect children and families. Parents rushing down the supermarket aisle with a child in tow should be credited with selecting products with fruit on the label. With precious little time, they make split-second decisions based on valuing their children's health. They shouldn't have to read the fine print to know whether a product with fruit in the picture has fruit in the package. That's not making the healthy choice the easy choice. As television personality Al Roker (who himself had stomach-reducing surgery) responded to our study on *Today*: "Wait a minute, my child eats this. I didn't know these were the ingredients."[14]

THE BLACK PANTHERS HAD IT RIGHT

The National School Meals Program is one of the most significant investments and opportunities in the United States to improve food access for children and prevent the various health consequences of malnutrition. What's not generally known about the program is that it was begun by the Black Panthers, a Black nationalist organization that grew out of Oakland,

California, in the 1960s. Acting in the interest of children and insisting that no child should be hungry, the Panthers began serving breakfast at St. Augustine's Church in West Oakland, and, before long, their efforts spread to chapters across the country. This outreach was of concern to the US government solely because of the people who were executing it: the Panthers' advocacy for Black pride, Black power, and gun-carrying rights made them a source of anxiety for the federal government, and their nutritional outreach—while likely confusing for federal authorities—became a target for co-opting.

Fearing that their influence and power might spread, and that the Panthers couldn't as easily be cast as fearsome radicals if they were known for organizing children's breakfasts, the government launched a new federal school food program in 1962; it has remained part of US policy for low-income children.[15] Of course, when the funding for school breakfast programs was made available to community groups, the Black Panthers were the obvious choice for Oakland, and for other cities, as the group best set up to provide them—but the federal government sought alternatives. In Oakland, churches joined together, forming a new group, the Council of Churches, with the promise they would receive the funding, not the Black Panthers. At least the principle of providing healthy breakfasts flourished.

Nearly a half century later, commitment to this program remains strong, and improved meals standards instituted in 2012 ensure that school-age children, particularly those in low-income communities, are receiving increasingly healthy meals at school.[16] At the same time, that connection between food and justice, which initially sparked the Black Panthers to take on school food, has led to more school gardens, farm-to-school programs, and activism in the community to ensure low-income children and children of color have access to healthy food.

This spark has more recently ignited a new form of community activism in West Oakland, where Elaine Brown, former chairwoman of the Black Panthers, has launched West Oakland Farms. A worker-owned collective that employs former inmates, the farm has turned a vacant lot into a thriving urban garden and community hub, selling fresh produce. "I'm not in the farm business," says Brown. "I'm in the business of creating opportunities for Black men and women who are poor and lack the education, skills, and resources to return to a community that is rapidly gentrifying without economic avenues for them in mind." The farm isn't just serving posh eateries; it's now providing fresh produce to the Oakland Unified School District's on-campus farmers' markets and soon to its newly opening central kitchen. The Black Panthers' passionate commitment to nourishing urban schoolchildren, empowering residents, and providing opportunities for self-determination in communities that have experienced disinvestment has come full circle.[17]

GROWING UP WITH A CHEF'S DAUGHTER

My great grandmother was a well-regarded chef at the Half Moon Hotel in New York. I never met her, but she had a big impact on my life: as a result of her cooking success, her daughter, my grandmother, felt inadequate and never cooked at all. My grandfather did all the real cooking.

That turned out to be lucky for me, because I spent a lot of time with my grandfather. I cooked alongside him from the time I was four or five, and it shaped my love of food. Tomato sauce with spaghetti, renamed "pasta" as food trends evolved, was, and still is, my comfort food. As much as eating it, I love the process of making it, chopping the mushrooms and onions and smelling the sweet aromas of garlic and tomatoes as they fill the room with anticipation for dinner. (That's where I learned to pop garlic into the hot olive oil the second guests arrive—everyone says, "Wow, dinner smells delicious.") It never occurred to me that a man was not supposed to cook—the great irony that you had to be a man to be a chef, but otherwise cooking was not manly.

Even the preparation, the shopping, was part of the ritual. At the small fruit stands in Coney Island, the vendors would carefully feel the tomatoes to make sure we got the ripest ones. It was important not to go the cheapest stores or the most expensive, either. Bargaining seemed to be part of the ritual, but my grandfather never did that, despite the fact that he was by no means wealthy. He knew the vendors' families and would never ask them to reduce their prices. As a result, the store owners simply acknowledged that he accepted their price by slipping a few extra fruits or vegetables into the bag. My grandfather would

hand me the bags, and I would proudly carry them back home. Years later,
cooking is natural for me and still a source of comfort.

My first food-related efforts in prevention were mostly focused
on its health-sustaining properties and whether or not it tasted delicious; to me those things were central to food's importance. Through
my involvement with the food movement over the decades since, I've
learned that the US food system also impacts both US and global well-
being in ways that may be less evident. The United Nations calculated
that livestock are responsible for nearly one-fifth of greenhouse gas
emissions, a larger share than cars and trucks. Like soda, meat consumes
vast amounts of fresh water and contaminates groundwater, while soak-
ing up robust federal subsidies. Sacrificing large tracts of rainforest to
meat production has also reduced the critical buffer needed to absorb
carbon dioxide and slow climate change. In addition, about one-third
of all arable land goes to animal fodder,[18] whereas using this land to cultivate whole grains and fresh produce for human consumption would
allow us to feed and sustain far more people—instead of producing
1 pound of meat, we could, for example, harvest 400 pounds of tomatoes or 350 pounds of potatoes.[19]

Global meat production has nearly tripled over the past forty years,
with people in the United States eating an average of 53 pounds *more* meat
annually than they did in 1950. Of course, that's an average, brought down
by people like me who don't eat meat, meaning others are taking in far too
much.[20] Yet the World Cancer Research Fund has recently recommended
people limit red meat consumption to no more than 18 ounces per week
to improve health.[21] Experts have also concluded that each 50-gram por-
tion of processed meat eaten daily increases the risk of colorectal cancer by
18 percent.[22] With the *increase* in US intake already hovering at the warning level, imagine the health risks when meat production doubles again
over the next forty-five years, as industry targets anticipate.

Food-related industries provide nearly 10 percent of US jobs and
contribute almost 5 percent to our gross domestic product,[23] yet,
cruelly, many of these jobs don't sustain families or rural communities. In fact, often farmers and farmworkers can't access the very food
they're growing. Facing constant economic challenges, farmers and
farmworkers are 3.6 times more likely to die of suicide than people

in other professions.[24] Agricultural workers and meat processors are some of the nation's lowest wage-earners, while farmers and workers alike also suffer from high rates of occupational injuries and chemical poisoning.[25,26,27]

The realities of our food system can feel overwhelming—too large and too entrenched to change all at once. But, as with so many big problems, communities and businesses are taking valuable steps to create the system we want and need. Indeed, it feels like the United States is at the beginning of a sea-change in its approach to food—with a swell of interest in seemingly old approaches, like farmers' markets, heirloom produce, and cooking from scratch, which benefit consumers and workers. As the movement has been building, its momentum and innovations have increasingly started to reshape government policies and industry practices in ways that ensure all people can enjoy the fruits of a healthier food system.

Frequently, the most successful strategies emerge at the local level first. Strategies such as making healthy food more affordable, getting junk food out of schools, passing soda taxes, and creating retail incentives like fresh-food financing are among the significant areas where the nation's policies are taking a strong position for health. Why is this more common on the local level? The answer is it is easier to be more specific in describing the changes needed and to reach the elected officials—without the extensive lobbying network and massive contributions to politicians. These are the beginnings of an ever-growing movement to shift the food system toward protecting personal and community well-being.

One of my favorite examples is the Healthy Food Financing Initiative (HFFI), a multisector partnership among departments of the treasury, agriculture, and health and human services. HFFI has created a seven-year program to eliminate "food deserts," by providing incentives for new grocery stores that offer fresh, affordable food in underserved areas. This initiative aims to lower rates of chronic diseases by making healthier foods accessible in lower resourced areas.[28] At the same time, by supporting economic vitality and creating thousands of jobs in rural and urban neighborhoods, the initiative offers people a way to sustainably raise their standard of living, helping them to thrive. This very successful initiative bubbled up from the local level to become state and then federal law.

THE PAINFUL IRONY OF HUNGER AND PLENTY

The United States has been called the breadbasket of the world, and yet in many low-income communities, food insecurity remains systemic. Even when individuals have enough for the moment, they feel at risk of being hungry in the days to come. Stretching the family food dollar often means going for the cheapest foods, leading consumers with low incomes to choices that perpetuate the cycle of hunger and illness. Even food stamps, designed to provide a minimum for those who need it, have become regulated to control who gets them and in what circumstances in irrational ways, often depriving some of those in greatest need. At a time in my life when I needed food stamps to make ends meet, I found the process humiliating and was asked a lot of questions that made me feel like a failure. And it's far worse now than it was for me then.

Organic food is one of the fastest growing segments of the food industry.[29] Yet organic food has generally been far more expensive at the cash register, partly because it is cultivated in smaller quantities with labor-intensive growing techniques, and it doesn't yet benefit from price supports. With wider cultivation and subsidies, this trend can quickly change (and of course is essential for our environment in the long term). Another type of product, *transitional crops*, which are not yet certified organic but are grown without the use of chemical pesticides, are becoming more widely available, offering a cheaper price point and a relatively better health value. With a deeper investment in sustainable methods, farmers' markets and other venues will be able to increase people's access to this segment.

Open-air markets are an everyday sight in most parts of the world. This isn't true in the United States, where farmers' markets are often recast as "bougie" (bourgeoisie) for being too expensive. Yet we're seeing a resurgence in this age-old tradition not only in high-wealth communities but in all neighborhoods. A large part of the growing enthusiasm for local food and farmers' markets began in wealthier neighborhoods, where people have more time and disposable income, but it's slowly expanding to every segment of the population, as community activists pursue strategies for increasing equitable food access. Some vendors are now equipped to take SNAP (food stamps) and WIC payments from low-income shoppers. Some offer flexible hours and better access via mass transit, greatly increasing diversity of shoppers.[30] Many of the farmers' markets have branched out, selling dried beans, other legumes, and assorted grains, nuts, and seeds at affordable prices. In Stockton, California, immigrant-rights groups are working with farmers' markets to finally establish a way for farmworkers to begin to access the very food they grow, which has been cruelly out of their reach.[31]

Pennsylvania's Fresh Food Financing Initiative, a recent community-driven effort to increase access to healthy food, is a recent example of how policy can effect change in this area. As residents of Philadelphia's low-income neighborhoods lived in food deserts (neighborhoods, typically low in median income, without access to grocery stores) and accordingly suffering from disproportionately higher levels of chronic disease, the city clearly was pressed to find a way to get full-service grocery stores into low-income neighborhoods. Community advocates from the Philadelphia Food Trust found a receptive politician, Dwight Evans, who helped marshal a variety of state resources and engage private investments. By 2009, the initiative had raised nearly $60 million in grants, funding both large and small grocery store owners to open or expand, including seventy-four supermarket projects in twenty-seven Pennsylvania counties. In addition to launching these new stores, the initiative created more than 5,000 jobs.[32] The effort has successfully bubbled up, spreading first to several other states and then becoming a seven-year federal initiative.[33]

THE HEALTH, FOOD, AND FARM BILL

The Farm Bill—our nation's primary legislation for shaping agricultural practices, subsidies, and national food policy—is one of the most sweeping and influential pieces of policy at any level of US government. The scope of the bill would be more aptly described as the Health, Food, and Farm Bill, as it would signal the root ways its decisions inform what the nation eats and, with it, what its disease profile will look like. Like many US laws related to agriculture, the Farm Bill is geared toward supporting corporate agribusiness; crop insurance, chemical fertilizers and pesticides, mechanization, livestock production, and other massive economies of scale have all traditionally benefited from the US Farm Bill.[34,35,36,37] These benefits have often come at the expense of consumers' health, the environment, and small to midsized farmers, as evidenced by the ever-reducing rural population and number of family-owned farms.[38]

A series of Farm Bill decisions over the years has taken its toll on the farmers who grow our fresh food sustainably. Leslie Mikkelsen, who launched our Prevention Institute's work on healthy eating, was invited to visit a midsized farm in Missouri to understand the farmer's perspective on the Farm Bill firsthand. Following in his father's footsteps, farm owner Rick had become a farmer out of love for the land and a passion for nourishing the nation. He shared a story illustrating how corporate power and federal farm policies constrict his choice of crops and undermine his ability to earn a decent living.

One year, Oswald tried to cultivate white corn used for masa to make tortillas—as he put it, "real food." He contracted with a grain elevator (a company that stores and sells grain) that typically bought "food grade" corn, which is actually not edible but is instead used for animal feed. Unlike growing food-grade corn, the effort to grow this crop was a risk. When the white corn crop failed around the region that year due to weather, horrifyingly, Oswald found he was expected to buy his contract back even though he hadn't accepted any money or even set a price. Worse, the wording of the contract enabled the elevator to set its own price without any hope of arbitration. In the past, the local owner of the grain elevator might have worked out a deal, allowing Oswald to simply carry the contract forward to the next year's production. Unfortunately, due to corporate competition and consolidation, the grain elevator was now owned by a large corporation, which was unwilling to make such accommodations. So the combination of corporate consolidation and the Farm Bill's prioritization of non-food colluded both against the farmer and against the consumer's interests in healthy food.

I started thinking about how the Farm Bill could better align with health several decades ago, when I met Nancy Milio, a nurse and leader in public health policy and education, who wrote about using our agricultural policy decisions to encourage health. Milio had developed and promulgated the notion that all areas of public policy affect health.

She pointed out that the decisions we make about food cultivation and the tools for encouraging what gets grown—our food policies, subsidies, corporate marketing practices, and environmental policies concerning resource ownership, availability, and cost—are health decisions, and we need to demand accountability for them, exercise our voice in determining them, and insist they align with health.

To illustrate this, she challenged the US decisions to invest in tobacco, oil seeds, and sweeteners, arguing that cultivating these has a destructive impact on our health. Her perspective was rejected here in her home country but embraced internationally, where she served as an analyst of food and nutrition policies in European countries and was celebrated by the international health community.

More recently, the health community—concerned about the rates of diabetes and other food-related chronic diseases—has become more actively engaged in the Farm Bill debate. Advocates for health, sustainable agriculture, and small to midsized farms are beginning to find common ground in promoting policy recommendations on the availability and affordability of healthy, whole foods that could address their multiple perspectives at once.[39,40]

A strong policy effort to support farmers and equitable food access is the Kentucky-based Community Farm Alliance (CFA). No-smoking laws had affected the livelihood of small to midsized farmers in the state. In the mid-1980s, many Kentucky farmers, who had grown tobacco for decades, were on the verge of losing their land. Reduced demand for tobacco, an influx of new residents, and increased real estate costs threatened to put many of the state's farmers out of business. In 1985, the CFA stepped in to establish a credit hotline, allowing thousands of farmers to stay on their land and make the transition away from tobacco. In 2000, the CFA won a huge victory that had been many years in the making, securing provisions from the state's Tobacco Settlement to support family farming and diversified farming practices. The CFA also worked with farmers to create farmer-owned distribution chains, cutting out the "middle man" and allowing growers to price their products more competitively.[41]

With strong measures in place to support sustainable farming, the CFA began to focus efforts on increasing demand. The group created two farmers' markets in low-income areas of Louisville, mutually benefitting the farmers and the consumers. These markets serve about 8,000 people annually, providing fresh fruits and vegetables to residents living in food deserts. The CFA also helped establish an incentive program for neighborhood corner store owners to help them offset the cost of carrying fresh, local foods.[42] Today, the CFA continues to bring together grassroots organizers to develop strong policies that support local and family farmers in Kentucky. Recently, the CFA successfully launched the Agriculture Legacy Initiative to support beginning farmers and the future of Kentucky family farming. CFA members—after more than thirty meetings with Kentucky legislators—passed a voluntary income tax check off to Kentucky food banks to purchase food directly from Kentucky farmers and integrated local food into the state capitol's cafeteria.[43] With CFA's leadership, more than two dozen pieces of legislation have been either passed or defeated in support of the farming community.[44]

In 2013 the Farm Bill was aptly renamed the Food and Farm Bill, reflecting the linkages between farm policy and food consumption and constituting a significant win for those who had struggled to make these connections better understood. The 2013 law also contained some wins regarding funding, including greater allocation for local, sustainable food production and increased supports allowing low-income people in the United States to better access fresh fruits and vegetables. It's early in terms of major change, but the policies represent a step in the right direction.

THE PUBLIC RIGHT TO KNOW

In the early 1990s I contributed to a food-labeling bill for California, one of the earlier efforts to give consumers accurate information about the foods they purchased. The food manufacturing lobby had resisted a national food-labeling bill that would disclose nutrients in foods (or lack thereof), so the attempt at a statewide bill seemed attainable. California was a large and lucrative food market, which precluded any food manufacturers from pulling products entirely in the face of new labeling requirements. With the Clinton presidency looming, manufacturers faced a Democratic chief executive with a record of consumer advocacy, and during the last days of the Bush administration they moved to get a national bill passed to preempt our more stringent California proposal. It was a necessary, though insufficient, step; it promoted the notion that industry accountability to the public was essential and that the public has a right to know what's in the food they buy.

~~Menu labeling~~ is a recent victory that has advanced industry transparency to the public. The goals were similar to those of the previous ~~food-labeling~~ endeavors—both to provide information that can help consumers make the healthy choice the easy choice and to create momentum for industry to change its practices. As eating out has changed from an occasional event to a very frequent occurrence—~~over 40 percent of every~~ ~~food dollar is spent outside the home~~—what people eat outside the home takes on much more importance in terms of overall well-being.[45] Despite vigorous industry resistance to disclosing ingredients to the public, community activists and public health leaders managed to pass menu labeling nationally as part of the 2010 Affordable Care Act (though enforcement has been repeatedly delayed due to industry concerns about the scope of the rule). While it's not a panacea, and we still need much broader changes, menu labeling has catalyzed product reformulation in some cases and kept the pressure on industry.

THE GOVERNATOR

When Arnold Schwarzenegger became governor of California in 2003, we in the California public health community knew he understood the importance of eating good food and being active—but we feared, given his success as a body builder, that he would see it all as individual responsibility. Shortly after his inauguration he held a summit on healthy eating and hosted all the TV stars he was connected to, from Dr. Phil to Dr. Oz. A coalition of our statewide partners, the Strategic Alliance, prepared a ten-point platform, knowing full well it would be overly assertive and out of step with conservative rhetoric. Surprisingly, the governor was responsive. By the time he left office, he had endorsed a state plan that reflected every element of the platform, enacted key legislation, and allocated funds to schools to make some of these policies a reality.

A key plank in our platform focused on schools, and perhaps one of the most impactful bills the governor signed was the strongest-in-the-nation school food standards, banning soda and the worst junk foods.[46] Prior to the legislation, spearheaded by the California Center for Public Health Advocacy, there were no restrictions on the products that the food and beverage industry could sell in schools, and children were treated as a captive audience for the worst of their products. In the years since, more states have implemented school food rules, culminating in 2010 with a national law to establish universal standards. Improvements like this have demonstrated measurable results: after California implemented its rule, the state's high school students took in 160 fewer calories per day, along with less sugar and fat, than their counterparts in other states that lacked similar standards.[47] The governor's action was another step in a long path toward ensuring healthy food in schools for all children.

TAKING ON BIG SODA

I was giving a talk in Mexico when its government made history, becoming the first nation to pass a soda tax—a breakthrough achievement. It was a hefty tax, at 10 percent per liter. With its people consuming a half liter of soda per day, Mexico had just surpassed the United States, with nearly a one-third obesity rate, the highest in the Americas. Serving a dual health effect, the tax proceeds were meant to provide drinking water in the schools. At a press conference there, I commented that this action would resonate widely, shifting cultural norms in the United States and across the Americas. One of the industry's most effective attacks on soda taxes in the United States is that they are discriminatory against people of color, because more Latinos and Black people have a low income and therefore pay a higher percentage of their income in such taxes. But the pride in Mexico as the first country to tax soda would seal, for Latinos, the conviction that standing up to an industry that was cavalier about diabetes was something they would be very proud of, and it would serve as a model to aspire to in the United States, thus weakening that cynical argument. The domino effect would start to build, as it did in our fight against tobacco, with Ecuador, Peru, and Chile investigating ways to decrease soda marketing and Barbados passing a 10 percent tax on sweetened beverages.

The United States has had a groundswell of activity that's also been gaining momentum. I recently supported the first successful US campaign to adopt a city soda tax in our neighboring city of Berkeley. Not surprisingly, beverage industry officials claimed such a tax would harm low-income, non-white populations most, because they spend the greatest proportion of their income and food budget on soda. As Eric Batch, a senior vice president of the American Heart Association, accurately countered, people of color and low-income people pay the *most* and get the *worst* in the current system pushing soda. Local leaders and advocates smartly preempted industry by working with residents in the communities suffering most from high rates of soda-related chronic diseases. A Black minister, whose son died of diabetes, was featured in a compellingly poignant campaign piece, part of highlighting many diverse endorsers of the measure. This personal tragedy helped Berkeley residents understand the real-life harm. In Berkeley, as in Mexico and now in many other places, we're starting to see soda take on the persona of tobacco. It's a powerful signal that norms are changing when it comes to sugar-sweetened beverages and the industry that produces them.

COOKING BY COLORS

Seeing purple cauliflower grow had a long-term influence on me, prompting me to think about food and colors. Years later, I resolved to do a cookbook based on this: Cooking by Colors. *I had no redeeming purpose in mind. I just thought it was fascinating to think about food in a new way and design some delicious combinations. Everyone I spoke to thought it was a great idea. If cooking is an art, color selection is part of it. When I refined my plan, I decided to start with monochromatic (one-color) cooking, and the same people reversed their opinion and universally rejected the idea. If color is interesting, it is because of its contrasts, diversity, and brightness. I had to agree, but I thought I had a really good idea for revealing contrast. As a fan of white-on-white painting like Rauschenberg's, I realized that gradients of color, or subtle differences within one color, made me much more attuned to nuances and distinctions. My proof of this and vindication was that virtually everyone, after saying that one color didn't work, soon proposed an interesting, inventive one-color recipe of their own creation. It made us all think and be creative, and that was the point.*

I called it the Experimental Dinner and invited staff. The word experiment *made some people nervous, but they came. Green was too easy, so
I prepared very simple brown and red dishes, using fresh, seasonal ingredients. The brown dish started with fresh mushroom fettuccine made by
my neighbor Eric at his little shop, Pasta Panificio, near Strawberry Creek.
I simply sautéed different kinds of brown mushrooms, like Shitake and
Cremini, in garlic and added a handful of almonds, which shimmered in
the pasta. Following this dish was a heated red salad, where I stir-fried red
onion with beets and, as it cooked, tossed roughly chopped radicchio into the
pan for about a half minute to make it softer. The olive oil I used to sauté
it became the salad dressing base. When it was prepared, I tossed in pome-
granate seeds and raspberries, adding balsamic vinegar to balance out the
oil and complete the dressing—delicious. After dinner, I asked: lemon sorbet
or chocolate cake for dessert?*

*At first, the Experimental Dinner may have seemed contrary to concepts
of good cuisine, but, in fact, it fit centrally with every culture's notion that food
matters—its taste, its look, the thought and preparation that go into a meal.
This was my new culture, a creative reconstruction of so many experiences and
places and a challenge of one color at a time. It got all of us thinking about the
food and the craft of preparation. There was much talking and laughing after
the initial nervousness and politeness subsided, furthering our connections as a
staff. This was the visceral experience of eating together, not noticing—though
it had been part of its essential construction—that it was grounded in values of
health, fairness, and environmental sustainability. Sustaining—there's no better way to appreciate that than over a great meal.*

[7]

INJURIES ARE NOT ACCIDENTS

RICKY

I was nine and noticed my mother looked sad when I came home one day. She was usually direct and generally comfortable with whatever needed to be said, so her reluctance to talk meant something was wrong. Then she told me that Ricky, a neighborhood kid my age, had been run over by a car while bicycling right around the corner from our house. In an odd way I was relieved; I knew my mother was going to say something serious, and at the time this didn't seem so bad. Ricky and I didn't play together much, and death didn't really upset me; I was too young to grasp its permanence. Besides, Ricky was a crossing guard at our school, and just that week he had threatened to give me a "summons" for crossing against the light, which I thought was stupid since there weren't any cars coming. I was still mad at him for being a stickler for the rules.

The devastation of Ricky's death didn't hit me in earnest until I saw his mother in the grocery store. I found myself backing away before she spotted me, imagining that if she saw me she would think of Ricky and get very sad. From then on, whenever I saw her I tried to avoid her, but sometimes she would see me, smile, and say hello. How could she be happy to see me and ask how I was doing? I couldn't bear to say I was okay or happy. I couldn't tell her about my day; it felt so small and trivial. What I felt most was shame—shame that I hadn't minded when I heard he died, shame that she seemed to like me, and shame to be alive when Ricky wasn't. Only then did I start to understand the permanence and poignancy of his death.

I grew up and left the area, and the tragedy faded from my mind—until the day I was speaking to law enforcement officials about their role in preventing traffic-related crashes. I was about to say that crashes and injuries could be predicted and prevented when an image of Ricky's mother flashed into my mind. It stopped me mid-speech. Suddenly, I connected Ricky's death to my prevention work. I had never thought about why he had been killed or what could have been done to prevent it. Maybe it was partly Ricky's fault for bicycling in the middle of the street, though we had all done so. Maybe the driver wasn't paying attention. I don't remember ever hearing anything about the investigation of the incident; it was grown-up talk, I guess. As a child, I took it for granted that things happened that were out of my control. Later, I realized that the grown-ups also seemed to have viewed the crash as fate or bad luck—an unhappy circumstance beyond anyone's control.

THE "A" WORD

It's common for people to use the word accident for car crashes, falls, burns, drownings, poisonings, and every other type of nonviolent injury. It's an unfortunate habit, because the word implies that injuries are simply happenstance, rare, and without pattern. The term blinds us to the frequency, predictability, and preventability of these injuries. Injuries are one of the largest disablers, killers, and expenses we face in our healthcare system, and they are a tragically early killer—the leading cause of death for people age one to forty-four[1]. Nevertheless, health research still focuses mainly on disease, as do most of our organized efforts to keep people well.

As a country, we're paying an enormous price—hundreds of billions of dollars each year in medical costs alone[2]—for our failure to treat injuries as preventable. Emergency departments and hospitals are clogged with injury victims, many of whom require costly and lengthy trauma care. This isn't just a US problem; in many countries internationally, there is a large and growing burden of injury-related deaths and costs, especially in countries where the average household income is low.[3] Personally, I've met far too many people who have experienced tragedies like the one Ricky's family suffered.

It's negligent not to apply the same energy we devote to preventing diseases to the often simpler task of preventing injuries. Research has given us a huge amount of knowledge and success in this area that we can expand upon rather than allowing unnecessary suffering to continue.

Rather than using the "A" word (accidents), injury specialists be using the term *unintentional injury* to describe injuries that happen without deliberation. Violence, including suicide and harm to others, was named *intentional injury*. As unwieldy as these terms are, they shift our associations and encourage a new mindset.

Saying *crashes* instead of *car accidents*, for example, is an easy way to refocus commonplace thinking and create a new mindset. The less fatalistic the language used for injuries, the easier it becomes to consider ways to prevent them.

Note that saying that injuries are preventable and predictable doesn't mean the events that caused them—the crash or the fire, for example— were planned. It means that factors in the environment and individual behavior can affect the likelihood of injuries and deaths occurring. Examples of these factors include uneven sidewalks, which can cause falls among older adults, and easy access to medicines, which can lead to poisonings in young kids. So actions such as investing in maintaining sidewalks and requiring childproof caps on medicine containers are important ways to prevent undue harm and save many lives.

Preventing harm is especially critical for communities that are less wealthy and face more discrimination because they have greater risk factors, such as ill-maintained roads, parks, and playground equipment and more stores that sell alcohol. These communities not only have fewer financial resources but also less political clout to effect policy and infrastructure change.[4] A disproportionately high number of people of color live in areas where disinvestment has increased their exposure to injury-causing conditions, so it's not surprising that they are at risk for more frequent and intense injuries in certain cases.[5] Of particular note, indigenous people including Alaskan Natives have the highest percentage of deaths due to unintentional injuries.[6]

Over the years, the prevention community has had enormous success in reducing and preventing certain types of injuries by identifying patterns, tracking back to the conditions that caused or exacerbated them, and taking actions to reduce the likelihood and severity of future injuries. An example is automobile safety, which has been declared one of the ten greatest public health achievements of the twentieth century.[7] Despite there being more cars, drivers, and miles traveled today than ever before, deaths and injuries from car crashes have declined remarkably over the past half century to record lows, thanks to important ~~changes in road design~~ and new ~~drunk-driving and seatbelt laws~~, among other changes.[8] These are national- and international-level policy changes that affect *all* communities, including disinvested ones.

Safety strategies save lives. This is, of course, the most important benefit, but they also provide some of the fastest and largest returns on investment. For example, requiring that infants ride in car seats, starting in the 1970s, saved money immediately, and these benefits have continued to accrue every year since. Every $46 ~~car seat~~ saves $140 in medical costs. In addition, that same car seat saves another $470 in future earnings, because parents do not miss work due to a tragic crash involving their child. Together, that's $610 in savings for each $46 seat—a ~~13 to 1 return on investment~~.[9]

Given the potential savings in lives, misery, and money, it's essential that we apply effective injury prevention strategies within every community in a systematic way. Doing so helps reduce pressure on healthcare and also fosters beneficial neighborhood conditions. However, far too often, when medical and policy leaders discuss health strategies and investments, they focus on advancing treatments, pharmaceuticals, and cures for *diseases*. Rarely do they think about injury prevention strategies, which are arguably far easier to achieve.

With many of the best unintentional injury strategies, such as requiring seatbelt use, it's simply a matter of applying our knowledge more broadly and systematically. ~~Some of the best solutions require no individual action at all: they are *passive* measures~~, like installing ~~air bags~~ or ~~antilock brakes~~, which reduce the likelihood and extent of vehicle-related injuries.

PENNY THE RIVETER

During World War II, tens of thousands of workers, most with little experience in building ships, poured into the Kaiser shipyards in Richmond, California, and throughout the Pacific Northwest. These workers produced ships at an unimaginable rate—one per week.[10] Working in the shipyards was more dangerous than most wartime industries, even riskier than making tanks, aircraft, and explosives.[11]

When Lucille "Penny" Price, an eighteen-year-old from Oakland, arrived in Richmond for her orientation, she heard a loud "beep, beep, beep" and a guide shout for everyone to duck. A crane's cable had snapped. Not everyone made it out of the way in time, and a deadly load of steel dropped on a group of workers. Price was lucky then, but she suffered numerous other injuries on the job—knife cuts, steel mesh in her eyes, and fiberglass down her neck and back. Once an explosion threw her off a deck and down a level, where she was severely burned and had her knee impaled. In spite of the heroic service she was giving to the country by doing this work, as a woman, Price faced both everyday job risks and even more egregious ones, due to discrimination and men's chauvinism. She was subjected to hostility and harassment. In one case, men pulled a ladder out from under her, cracking her ribs, and in another instance, they rattled a plank where she stood six stories up, nearly killing her.

The experiences of people like Price made the US industrialist Henry J. Kaiser realize that, to keep his workers healthy, meet war production demands, and protect his bottom line, he had to make the work environment safer. Walking through the shipyards, he discovered how to improve design and workflow patterns, especially in relation to falls and swinging cranes, which were the biggest sources of injury. Eleanor Roosevelt, a great prevention advocate, was thinking along the same lines. When she and President Roosevelt visited the shipyards, paying tribute to the Kaiser war effort as well as its new medical program, she asked, "What is your plan for preventive care?" [12] Soon after, the US Maritime Commission began working in tandem with Kaiser, implementing a more comprehensive safety prevention program that reduced disabling injuries by nearly one-half within a year.[13]

Workplace safety efforts have clearly increased since World War II, but the issue remains only partially addressed, despite people spending so much time on the job. Latinos in particular have the highest rates of fatal occupational injuries, with particularly high rates in the agriculture/forestry/fishing and mining industries.[14,15] Supporting injury prevention broadly and instituting workplace wellness initiatives makes sense from a health perspective. Just as important, businesses can lower health-care costs, absenteeism, and workers' compensation claims.[16] Given that private businesses today pay 20 percent of the $3 trillion national expenditure on healthcare in the United States, smart corporations are increasingly realizing the value of investing in workers' health and safety.[17] After all, workplace wellness programs alone can save businesses $6 for every $1 invested—half saved in medical expenses and the other half in costs relating to absenteeism.[18] Unfortunately, businesses often prioritize making a short-term profit over people's health, inaccurately calculating the full expense of illness and injury and failing to capture the savings from health.

WHAT INDIVIDUALS CAN DO

A reporter once phoned me and asked what the five most common home injuries are, what room in the house is most dangerous, and what a family can do to prevent injuries. The bathroom might seem to be the most problematic, she reasoned, due to its hard surfaces, water, electricity, and potentially toxic substances. In reality, I explained, the most dangerous room depends largely on the ages of the people living in the house. For young kids, drowning, suffocation, poisoning, and falls are top concerns, and injuries overall are their leading cause of death. For adults, prescription drug overdoses, falls, and fires are some of the most significant issues—and with prescription drugs, there is a mix of intentional and unintentional consumption. After explaining this, I tried to talk about violence, including suicide, which is also a common and serious threat in homes. The reporter simply said, "Oh, that's not what I mean." It's common for reporters to ask what individuals can do to prevent unintentional injuries. They ask the same questions about healthy food and alcohol use. While this may be a good way to frame a short news story and create an easy checklist for readers, individual action is only a small piece of the solution. In reality, and as discussed earlier, the environments in which people live and the products that are available and marketed to them are much more likely to harm or help protect them. To truly safeguard individuals, families, and communities, it's important to consider what builders, manufacturers, marketers, and policymakers can install upstream to create an environment of health and safety. For example, when architectural design incorporates handrails and step treads, the likelihood of a person falling on the stairs drops dramatically. When that design includes stairway landings, the impact from falls that actually occur is reduced. Policymakers can help ensure that safety features like these become mandatory. As I told the reporter, one of the most important actions people can take is to talk about the need for safety measures to their congressional representatives and influential governmental entities, such as the Consumer Product Safety Commission and the National Highway Traffic Safety Administration.

FALLS

The unthinkable tragedy of children falling from windows in high-rise apartments sparked an ongoing safety campaign in New York City. This tragedy occurred most frequently in low-income tenements, which had no air-conditioning, prompting people to leave windows wide open during the summer. In the 1970s, outraged residents and advocates demanded window guards, a simple, inexpensive, and effective solution—but building owners didn't want to spend the money to install them. Unfortunately, the fire department quietly backed the building owners, concerned that window guards could hamper rescues. Reaching a compromise, the city put window guards in all low-income, high-rise buildings in Harlem and the Bronx only. Once they were in, falls from these apartments virtually ceased. Most falls in the city then happened in higher-income areas, and the city was quick to respond, passing a universal window guard law that most other large cities have since adopted.[19,20]

Older adults are also highly vulnerable to injuries. In their case, the biggest risk is falling, often just while walking, due to their impaired balance and vision and diminishing strength.[21] Falls are more damaging and costly in this age group due to greater frailty: in the United States in 2013, medical expenses for older adult falls alone were $34 billion, not including costs like family caregiving.[22] Once people are injured, they are often less active and less able to care for themselves, so each injury has a potential multiplier effect, increasing the likelihood of other concerns. And with the number of people age sixty-five and over expected to double in the United States within the next forty years, this is a critical time to invest in preventing falls.[23]

Increasing safe physical activity among older adults helps prevent falls by improving strength and balance and also can improve the chronic conditions that many older adults face, like heart disease and diabetes. Home modifications, like installing ~~window guards, railings, nightlights~~, and ~~slip-free rugs~~, play an important role in preventing falls and injuries at all ages, as does incorporating safety features and making needed repairs in municipal buildings and on the streets. One great inexpensive and simple solution to reducing falls in seniors is wearing ~~sneakers with Velcro closures, which eliminates tripping on shoela~~ces. Fall prevention strategies yield financial benefits as well as health benefits. For example, the Tai Chi: Moving for Better Balance exercise programs have been shown to save more than $5 for every $1 spent.[24]

MAKING MEDICINE SAFER

My young nephew was sick, and I reached for the aspirin. "No," he said, "I want Motrin. It tastes like cherry candy." While I understand that candy flavoring encourages children to take needed medication, it worries me that the sweet taste of some medicines can lead to kids wanting to consume too much. In fact, many children were poisoned from over-the-counter drugs and dietary supplements before manufacturers were forced to develop childproof caps.[25] These caps are undoubtedly helpful, but they still don't eliminate risk. My seven-year-old nephew could put together effortlessly a Lego game that was supposedly for nine- to twelve-year-olds. Even with childproof caps, when medication is in the house at arm's length, it suggests a lot of trust in the notion that kids won't have the skills to open childproofed packaging.

The Poison Prevention Packaging Act of 1970 required medicines to be childproofed, and the number of poisonings fell sharply.[26] Before then, people died unnecessarily while drug manufacturers resisted this safety change. The solution was straightforward and the costs not that significant, but it took community outcry to break down the barriers of industry.

Even with the change in packaging, poisoning is currently the leading cause of unintentional injury death, just surpassing car crashes.[27] Of course, many other dangerous household products, such as bleach, cleansers, and antifreeze, also cause poisoning. Black and Native American children have a much higher rate of poisoning than other races—another example of unjust health disparities that points to other, larger disparities in environment.[28]

I met a woman at one of my talks, and she told me a very sad story. Her adult daughter had been going through a tough time and couldn't sleep. After drinking heavily one night, she went to the medicine cabinet in her boyfriend's house, where she found lots of old prescription drugs from his entire family. The young woman overdosed and never woke up. The drugs seemed an accessible "solution"—far more so than mental health or substance abuse services that could have enabled her to deal with her concerns. I was very moved and didn't know how to respond but vowed that I would do something.

I learned that overdoses from prescription drugs were (and still are) becoming more common; in 2015, they were a bigger problem than overdoses from illicit drugs. So why don't manufacturers and pharmacies take unused or expired medications back, I wondered? Instead, these medications linger in people's homes as potentially deadly enticements and show up in communities' water supplies due to improper disposal in toilets or household garbage. If newspapers and bottles can be recycled, recycling drugs should also be a standard requirement.

A year after I met the woman whose daughter died, I worked alongside Nate Miley, a representative on the Board of Supervisors for Alameda County, where Prevention Institute is located. Together and with many others rallying, we supported passage of the first law in the nation to create a drug take-back program. Due to industry resistance, the board created a "study period" before taking up the law. It was inconceivable to me that the pharmaceutical industry—which cites its profit margins to court stock market investments—repeatedly claimed it couldn't afford the take-back program.

In the end, thanks to the collaborative efforts of public, civic, and private stakeholders, Alameda County created a successful safe medication disposal program.[29] In 2013, 14 tons of household-generated pharmaceutical waste were collected.[30] Take-back programs like this don't solve the whole problem of drug overdoses or suicides, but they are one important step that has other benefits as well.

IF CIGARETTES DIDN'T STAY LIT

My colleague Andrew McGuire has changed how fires are viewed in this country, bringing to light the high number of children who suffer burns from ~~flammable sleepwear.~~ Motivated by his own experience being badly burned as a child, he became a tireless advocate, catalyzing a grassroots movement to prevent other children from being burned.[31] He also made an Emmy award–winning movie on the subject.[32] I remember McGuire's heroic determination as he flew weekly from the West Coast to Washington, DC, to testify in front of a congressional committee investigating fire safety. He had the perseverance and savvy to get sleepwear regulations changed.

McGuire also took on the problem that cigarettes did not extinguish on their own. It is known that many fires start and homes burn down when people fall asleep—in many cases intoxicated—with lit cigarettes.[33] Historically, cigarettes remained lit because the manufacturers design them so the porosity of the paper purposely keeps them ignited, so they burn more quickly, including when set down.[34] McGuire helped expose this practice as well as the industry's successful, yet undisclosed, development of self-extinguishing or "fire-safe" cigarettes. While there's no such thing as a "safe" cigarette, it's important to minimize the fire hazard from cigarettes—and save lives—by ensuring that they are self-extinguishing. Cigarette companies falsely claimed they had no solution, but endless hearings finally prompted them to admit they had the technology in hand to ensure that cigarettes self-extinguished. McGuire's work eventually led to all fifty states adopting identical laws mandating fire-safe cigarettes.[35]

Why does it have to take so many tragedies to gain mainstream attention and change regulations? It shouldn't require people like McGuire needing to fly across the country every week to participate on a national committee just to accomplish the obvious: establish regulations that decrease the deaths caused by unsafe products. And despite the fact that fire-safer cigarettes were doable and needed, it took decades for the regulations to be incorporated across the nation, due to industry chicanery and resistance. How many more people died during those long weeks while the committee was hearing testimony or during the many years until the safety standards were fully established across the nation? Who are the people who want to support corporations that supply products that bring so much suffering to families? It's fortunate that we have community advocates like McGuire, and further battles can and need to be won to make our environments safer and healthier.

DANGEROUS WATERS

A child drowning is beyond a parent's worst nightmare. My colleague, Nadina Riggsbee, lived this nightmare when she got a call that her children, under the care of a babysitter, had fallen into a backyard swimming pool. Riggsbee rushed home to find one of her children dead and the other so seriously affected that he has been on life support for more than three decades.

Despite her personal agony, Riggsbee has become a heroic advocate for four-sided fencing around swimming pools. It's been a predictably difficult and poorly funded, community-by-community battle. As with childproofing medications, the solution is straightforward, but businesses with overwhelming financial interests have stymied its adoption and, so far, despite the lives that could be saved, there has been minimal success. Having someone like Riggsbee tell her story can create the political traction needed locally. But we certainly don't want to wait for such devastating stories in every locale—and for people with the courage, charisma, and determination of Riggsbee—in order to have success.

When advocates like Riggsbee challenged swimming pool manufacturers to require four-sided fences, the manufacturers spent lobbying time and money opposing the measure because it would increase cost and, they feared, diminish sales. They argued that full fencing would infringe on the rights of people without children and others who didn't want a visual barrier separating their home and pool. Following the "beware of the nanny state" playbook, the industry and its lobbyists invoked concerns about freedom, when, in fact, they were protecting their financial interests. So whose freedom were they really defending? And what about responsibility?

With Riggsbee leading the way and an injury prevention coalition in support, we countered that pools were sold with houses as permanent equipment, so safety features had to be built in, or future families and guests with children would be at undue risk. We also noted the high costs of care for the

5,000 children who survive drownings each year, ranging from $75,000 for initial emergency room treatment to $500,000 annually for long-term care.[36] Imagine how many lives could be saved with that money if it were used to support prevention.[37]

Swimming pools are one part of the drowning problem, while streams, lakes, and oceans are another. I learned that drowning is a huge concern in Hawaii, for example, when I went there for meetings with the Keiki Injury Prevention Coalition. "Keiki" means "child" in Hawaiian,[38] though it's a word that embodies a greater sense of love and care than the English equivalent. After several work days with the coalition, I was looking forward to enjoying some good snorkeling, and Ralph Goto, the chief lifeguard on Oahu,[39] offered to show me around.

It soon became clear that Goto and his colleagues take drowning quite seriously. At Hanauma Bay, a special coral reef preserve that's famous for snorkeling, we stopped to meet some of his lifeguards. Goto was anxious to share his work and pointed out the creative signage he had meticulously designed to cue inexperienced visitors to the safe areas and deter them from the dangerous sites. He also demonstrated a one-of-a-kind rescue boat his team had made specifically for the Hawaiian waters. The breathtaking rescues he shared via video left me awestruck. Goto had every angle covered. While prevention was his primary focus, he was clearly ready for rescues when needed. In addition, he had created an effective airline video that stated, "Welcome to Hawaii, and be cautious."

Our next stop, Sunset Beach, was an especially alluring one, with a beautiful name and a captivating view. It drew all the tourists who couldn't get into Hanauma Bay, which limits visitors to protect the reefs. The lifeguards knew the terrain and the trouble spots and could anticipate the swimmers' needs and potential problems. Unlike traditional lifeguards up on a perch, Hawaii's were down in the sand proactively assessing the situation. Identifying those who seemed unfamiliar with snorkeling and the beach, they would quickly warn these swimmers and offer advice.

Sunset Beach has a very strong, unpredictable undertow and a shallow shelf. Sometimes people are seriously injured there—some even break their necks. Ralph asked my advice on this, and I suggested they rename it Quadriplegic Beach to convey a "subtle" safety message. Needless to say, my idea wasn't met with much enthusiasm. I imagine the hotels and tourist bureau, which help pay for the lifeguards' work, wouldn't find it appealing. I had succeeded in convincing myself, however, and chose not to swim at this beach.

Ralph worked hard and smart to change the norm for how lifeguards approached their job. He also succeeded in upgrading their salaries, benefits, and status, which earned them more respect and helped him retain skilled staff. What impressed me most was when one lifeguard said to me—with no prompting from Goto—"Our job is prevention." These are the kinds of norms and actions that save lives.

THE BARNES DANCE

When I was fourteen years old, Henry Barnes became the traffic commissioner of New York City. It's amazing that I noticed this as a fourteen-year-old and still remember it—a sign of Barnes's ability to attract attention. He said that Manhattan's traffic was unacceptable; he would end the gridlock. Everyone's life would improve, he said, because he would reduce commute and delivery times an average of thirty minutes per trip. People generally think there's no way to change traffic—it's "just the way it is." Not Henry Barnes.

A big part of his solution was to make nearly all of Manhattan's streets one-way. The narrower side streets had been one-way for years, but the wider avenues were two-way.[40] Barnes realized that if an avenue were six cars wide and four of these lanes were for parking and double-parked vehicles, all the other traffic had to squeeze into one lane in each direction. Every time a vehicle made a left turn, traffic came to a standstill. With a one-way avenue, several of those same six lanes could accommodate traffic flow, and left turns would be swift and safer without oncoming traffic.

Barnes thought about pedestrian safety, too. He zeroed in on Broadway and 42nd Street; what better place to get attention for a daring innovation than Times Square? With heavy cross-traffic and cars turning, it was hard for pedestrians to stay safe. So he added a new segment in the traffic-light rotation that was for pedestrians only. With traffic stopped, pedestrians could cross horizontally and diagonally. The press aptly named this the Barnes Dance.[41]

How I wanted to be Barnes! Such simple, intuitive innovations, and they worked! I can vouch for the fact that he did indeed cut travel time across Manhattan by thirty minutes during rush hour, just as he had promised. Predictably, there were far fewer crashes and injuries after these citywide changes went into effect.[42,43]

It's interesting that Barnes's number-one priority wasn't even safety; his main objectives were to move traffic more efficiently, save people time, and reduce stress and frustration. He was focused primarily on the convenience of auto occupants, but his work was critical for pedestrians as well. Barnes gave New Yorkers more time, convenience, and safety in one stroke.

THE PROBLEM WITH BLAMING THE DRIVER

When I started my career in prevention, I looked into injuries occurring in the small city of Pittsburg, California. I created a map with pushpins indicating where serious crashes had occurred. The news wasn't good, as many of the crashes were on School Street, near the city's high school. I went straight to the administrator responsible for traffic, and, showing him the findings, I said, "We have to slow traffic at that spot to reduce the number of crashes." To my surprise, he told me that his job was to do the opposite—to make traffic move faster and to minimize automotive congestion.

The notion of slowing down traffic, even in the heart of town, is often not welcomed. Too many people in the United States maintain that the car is king, and in the everyday rush to get places faster, speed is both a luxury and a goal. Unfortunately, most traffic safety policy still mirrors a general fascination with the car, with success measured by the drop in auto-related injuries per mile traveled, rather than a reduction in the number of auto-related injuries altogether. As traffic safety expert Dinesh Mohan describes it, that makes as much sense as saying we are having success with malaria because we are reducing the number of deaths per mosquito—even at times when the number of overall deaths is increasing.

The introduction of the automobile created a massive new safety burden in the United States and worldwide. To divert attention from the overarching safety risks, auto manufacturers have become adept at attributing crashes to *driver error.* Along the way, they have dodged their own responsibility and opposed obviously effective safety mechanisms, such as seatbelts, air bags, and better side panels and bumpers.

Dr. William Haddon, the first head of the National Highway Safety Administration, achieved his position by advocating for effective traffic injury prevention strategy.[44] He designed a grid to analyze all the elements involved in a crash—not just drivers, but equipment, road design and condition, as well as medical response before, during, and after a crash.[45] This tool, called the Haddon Matrix, promoted a new mindset. People began to realize that injuries can occur even when a driver is careful. There are ways to make outcomes less severe when driver error is part of the equation as well. My colleague Ian Roberts states this issue of driver error versus broader responsibility creatively. Clapping his hands, he asks, "Where does the sound come from? Neither the left nor the right hand makes noise alone; it comes from the interaction."

STREETS BELONG TO EVERYONE

My colleague Sandra and I were driving on a stretch of Buford Highway near Atlanta that's notorious among our fellow injury prevention advocates. We could tell from the billboards and storefronts that this area, which is just outside the upscale Atlanta suburbs, was home to low-income Latino and Vietnamese families. As we traveled late one evening, we saw many older adults and mothers with young children walking in a dirt footpath that shouldered the road and served as a makeshift sidewalk. The occasional bus stop was nothing more than a pole in the dirt, with people squatting on rocks by the roadside, waiting. The hilly terrain limited visibility in many key areas, though this didn't slow the rushing traffic. We had to dodge careening taxis and private vans that were competing to fill the high demand for transportation in an area where residents were too poor to afford cars.

Neighborhood stores, markets, and restaurants lined the road, but without crosswalks or stoplights, sometimes for up to a mile, the only way people could access them was to walk, or rather run, "seven lanes of fear." The "middle suicide lane," as it's ominously called by locals, was swelling with people trying to manage kids and parcels as they waited for a break in traffic to attempt the second half of the crossing. People who live in communities like this have to defy death many times a day just to go to work and school and live their lives.

In the 1980s, pedestrians in New York City faced similar problems along Queens Boulevard, where a particular intersection had become among the city's deadliest. Media dubbed the street "Boulevard of Death" and "Killer Boulevard." Richard Retting, safety office director in the transportation department, began identifying problematic patterns. He first discovered that most of the victims were older and unable to cross the street within the time allowed before the light changed. He also noted that residences were all on one side and commercial areas on the other side, just as they are on Atlanta's Buford Highway, making the dangerous crossing a necessity. The road had obviously been designed with only cars in mind, without consideration for pedestrians. "One only needs to see the roadway itself to realize something is terribly wrong here. Disaster is waiting to happen," said Retting.[46]

Retting met with traffic officials, older adult residents, and community leaders, and together they pushed for comprehensive change. Most important, his team lengthened the time for the walk signal, made the countdown box more visible, and illuminated roadway markings. They worked with law enforcement to reduce speeding and held safety presentations at senior centers.[47] These improvements represented an important milestone in acknowledging that it's important to safeguard *all* people's lives, including vulnerable ones. Like much of injury prevention, none of these changes was hard to figure out. It was simply a question of attention and political will. Of course, it cost some money initially, but far, far less than the financial and personal costs of the injuries and deaths that would have occurred. After the project was completed, the number of annual pedestrian deaths predictably plunged.[48]

Once communities have identified what needs to be done, they should implement these safety measures *everywhere*—in cities and rural areas, in rich and poor neighborhoods. Press coverage of poor immigrant families at risk in Georgia is paltry compared to the media attention New York gives its older residents. Georgia also spends less than 1 percent of its $2 billion in transportation funding on pedestrian safety.[49] This dribble has gone to wealthier Atlanta suburbs, where road design has been improved, with sufficient crossings, medians, and infrastructure changes to help calm traffic. It's time to ensure safety for the rest of the community as well.

Streets belong to everyone. Where they have been co-opted as *roads*—oriented toward cars and trucks—it's because decision-makers with vested interests in the auto industry exercise a mentality that fails to consider how vehicles affect the physical and community environments of non-drivers. A big step in lessening our cultural dependence on cars is constructing environments in which all modes of travel are safe, including walking, biking, navigating a wheelchair, pushing a walker or stroller, and traveling safely to and from public transit. People are already walking and biking more than in recent years, but bicyclists and pedestrians suffer disproportionately from traffic injuries in the United States. In fact, the number of pedestrian fatalities is equivalent to a jumbo jet crashing monthly.[50] Polls have consistently shown that *many* more people would walk regularly if they had access to safe, designated paths.[51]

I like the term "completing the streets," which refers to design that considers all the different modes of getting around.[52] Traffic calming is one aspect that leads to friendlier streets. It uses subtle design changes and aesthetic enhancements to slow down cars and make all forms of mobility safer and more pleasurable. I've seen cities where bike lanes are separated from other traffic, so cyclists ride safely using the line of parked cars as a natural barrier. In other cases, cyclists ride with traffic but wait at the light in designated boxes at the head of the queue, where they are more visible to drivers. It's a subtle way of saying bikes go first. More and more communities are using blinking lights on the ground at crosswalks and are moving crosswalks away from the corners a bit, so drivers can better focus on right turns and on seeing pedestrians. Changes like these are occurring slowly, but they provide hope that ever-more innovative solutions can be applied to saving lives.[53]

INJURIES ARE NOT ACCIDENTS

While working for a county health department, I printed a bumper sticker that read, "Injuries are not accidents." My colleagues and I convinced our county government to order that it be placed on every municipal vehicle, though we never expected to see it on road-building equipment, tractors, and even lawn mowers. I put one on my car as well. Sometimes I'd notice people come up to my car to read the small print on the bumper sticker, making funny expressions as they tried to figure out what it meant. Some looked completely bewildered, others walked away pondering, and a few brightened as new ideas dawned on them. At Prevention Institute, we've reprinted the bumper stickers saying "Injuries are not accidents. They are predictable and preventable."

I have made community safety one of my urgent prevention goals. I like the two-for-one benefit—the same changes to the environment that increase safety will also alleviate other health problems. For example, making areas more pedestrian-friendly encourages physical activity, which reduces chronic diseases like diabetes. It also lowers the use of cars, which decreases air pollution and its associated respiratory diseases. Here again, we see how a good solution solves multiple problems.

[8]

STAY SAFE

THE FULL-SIZED SHOTGUN

Walking home just before dark one night, I caught sight of two men talking. Their interaction seemed tense, but I didn't react quickly enough to the cues. It was a holdup at gunpoint. When the robber saw me, he thought he'd get a second haul. Before I knew it, I was looking into the barrel of a full-sized shotgun. Not sawed off—full size. Then he pushed it into my chest. He took my wallet and watch, threw my keys into the nearby bushes, and disappeared. For a long time after this incident, I was afraid to go home after dark. I was afraid to go to sleep. I kept reliving that moment of terror.

It was months before I shared this story, except with my closest friends. I felt embarrassed, as though it had been my fault. I was ashamed that I still felt scared. Then one day, when I was giving a talk on violence prevention, I described this incident in response to a question. My voice quivered. A parent whose son had been shot thanked me for talking about my experience from the podium. "It validates our feelings and humanizes every one of us," she said. Ever since then, I often share this story when I speak about violence. My voice nearly always shakes. I know there are people in every audience who have suffered far more serious tragedies and wounds, and I've learned how critical it is to bring these experiences out into the open to diminish feelings of shame and stigma, as we try to come to terms with violence.

Reporters sometimes ask for my thoughts on incidents they call "senseless violence," knowing I've been extensively engaged in helping communities develop strategies for preventing violence. It's important for us to understand what's behind this question. Is "senseless violence" truly senseless? When reporters use this term, they're actually talking about violence that seems *callous*, with no apparent motive. Medically, a callous is not a sudden wound but the result of a more constant irritation—a wearing down. Likewise, violence is often an outcome of a systematized wearing down of communities, families, and individuals—by economics, inequality, trauma, social norms and systems, and power relations. Violence is preventable, but it's not often understood that way.

This leads to the question: When is violence perceived to make sense? I don't know that it ever does, but when it's portrayed that way, it often follows prejudicial lines of thought. For many people, the wealthier and whiter the victim and perpetrator, the less sense the violent act seems to make. By contrast, the poorer and darker-skinned the victim and perpetrator, the more accepted the violent encounters. Too many US residents view violence as normal in disadvantaged neighborhoods, where deteriorated living conditions jeopardize health and safety. When people say, "That's just the way it is there," as though the violence were inevitable, it further marginalizes communities and individuals whose lives have systemically been devalued. What does it say about US society when for people of a certain race the impact of violence is seen as acceptable? It says a lot about the assumptions and biases in this country, ones that impact people's level of outcry and demand for solutions.

The murders at schools in Columbine, Colorado, in 1999, and in Newtown, Connecticut, in 2012, were horrific, and the breadth of the suffering staggered the nation, lying heavily on everyone's hearts. These incidents created an intense media spotlight that captured many people's attention about the existence of violence and prompted important conversations about the potential solutions, especially gun regulations and the need for mental health services.

An extremely poignant moment in the aftermath of the Columbine school massacre came when a white woman, whose child had been killed, said to reporters, "I didn't know this happened to real people." I can't fathom the pain she was experiencing, but there was incredible pathos in her statement. It shows that she never expected violence in her community—and the rest of the country responded with shock and attention. It's alarming that the same compassion and demand of action isn't shown for the disproportionately high levels of violence experienced by children of color, children living in poverty, and immigrant and LGBTQ children.[1] It's forgotten that they are real people who are experiencing and suffering from violence—when they shouldn't be and don't have to be.

Every act of violence is unacceptable, part of the same tragedy that claims more than 30,000 lives every year in the United States[2,3] In the United States, homicide is the second leading cause of death among youth and the primary cause among Black youth.[4] It's appalling, unacceptable, and totally preventable.

Violence is such a national epidemic, in fact, that each catastrophe seems a bit less shocking to those not involved—accepted as a fact of life that's sorrowful but expected, without addressing what leads to violence or how it affects people's lives, livelihoods, and community experiences. Many interwoven aspects of US culture, social norms, and living conditions contribute to the likelihood that violence will occur. Also, for those with options, violence and the fear of it influence where we choose to live, work, learn, and play. For people who don't have the same options, the presence of violence influences the opportunity to work, play, learn, or shop at all. But we know this can change and many communities are demanding such change. Preventing violence is simply a question of political will, which must catch up to the need and demand.

Other wealthy nations experience a fraction of the murders that occur in the United States.[5] Oddly, this should give us hope. It means that the violence we see is clearly not normal, biological, or necessary—*and it is preventable*. If we insist on having safe air travel, we should also expect our homes, schools, and communities to be safe. Building on decades of learning and discoveries from my own and colleagues' work, I can say that we now know what to do to prevent a good deal of violence. We've worked with cities across the country where rates of street violence have been reduced up to 50 percent.[6,7] We can begin to anticipate causes and create solutions in our neighborhoods, altering the conditions and attitudes that encourage violence—*before* more children are killed anywhere.

A COALITION IS NEEDED

As director of prevention for Contra Costa County, I launched one of the nation's first coalitions to prevent violence, the Alternatives to Violence and Abuse Coalition (AVAC). This created as much of a stir—and perhaps more skepticism—among many county staff as when I had started working on no-smoking laws. People knew violence was the leading cause of death among youth in our county, but wasn't it a police issue? How could agencies outside of law enforcement and criminal justice help secure community safety? Besides, what did violence prevention have to do with health? Sure, emergency rooms were backed up and left holding the bag, especially for the numerous uninsured victims of violence, but health's role was patching people up in the aftermath. There was no pill to prevent violence and no treatment for its causes. And while no-smoking laws were just taking hold, laws against violence were well established, though obviously not effective enough. Even if public health did have a role, the notion of creating a *partnership* to prevent violence was still fairly unusual. For the most part, individual agencies and community groups—such as the Suicide Intervention Agency, the Battered Women's Shelter, the Child Abuse Prevention Agency, the Alcohol and Drug Abuse Council—ran their own programs and educational campaigns.

Several leaders of these agencies approached me with the idea of our working together. Seeing the success of the smoking-prevention work and the outcomes from strong partners joining forces, they expressed confidence that collaboration among agencies that address various types of violence could be critical. They weren't quite sure of the precise outcomes desired, but they were frustrated at how difficult it was to change the frequency of violence and wanted to explore new solutions.

Some of the initial collaborative opportunities seemed straightforward. For example, people calling the suicide prevention hotline might be struggling with a range of issues, such as domestic abuse, bullying, or alcohol use, and hosting discussions in workplaces about women's safety might equally raise concerns about domestic violence or substance abuse, so the staff of different agencies needed cross-training on how to best support these concerns. Further, understanding each other's challenges and strategies enhanced everyone's work. But in sharing information, we also hoped to more deeply discover the underlying conditions that make violence so entrenched in US culture and so seemingly hard to eradicate.

As we looked more closely at the different forms of violence and how they played out in communities, we began to realize that all forms of violence had commonalities and were interrelated. People experiencing (or perpetrating) domestic violence likely also had abused children in their household or had been abused as children. Studies were showing nearly all the people on death row had been abused and/or sexually assaulted as children.[8] Violence was emerging as cyclical, with multiple effects on those experiencing it. We wanted to discover the *common roots* of these different forms of violence.

It also quickly became clear that most of the organizations in our coalition focused on what was considered personal or "family" matters, such as substance abuse, child abuse, domestic violence, and suicide. No group dealt with street violence, defined as violence among nonfamiliar individuals. We knew certain cities had particularly high rates of homicide and assault within low-income "minority" populations, as they were called at the time. Yet none of the violence intervention and prevention groups directly addressed this significant problem, and virtually none had its primary offices in those cities, which were among the county's most densely populated.

Realizing the police were the primary group attending to street violence, we concluded that for too long we'd relied on tracking down and punishing offenders, which resulted in an immense criminal justice and incarceration system without reducing the rates of violence. While few disagree that policing is an important piece of addressing violence, an approach focused primarily on criminal justice is insufficient, ineffective, costly, and inhumane—as after-the-fact intervention comes too late to prevent suffering and trauma. Worse yet, it reinforces the cycle of violence, offering few options or alternatives. We understood that the realities of violence begged for strategies beyond traditional efforts that blame and punish. None of the groups could take the lead on addressing street violence alone, as they each had a different mandate, history, and expertise. This required a more comprehensive approach with cooperation between multiple partners. Our coalition also realized it was essential to further partner with organizations and advocates based in, and fully representing, the communities most affected by this violence. Clearly, we needed prevention-focused collaboration and a community-wide strategy, which our prevention program staff readily facilitated.

Our effort to understand each other's approaches and goals was unusual. We created opportunities for mutual advocacy and increased success, because we could speak to these issues with one collective voice. AVAC also recognized early on the interconnections between and need to attend to all forms of violence, including street violence, as a significant health issue. We hadn't yet developed comprehensive strategies for addressing the underlying causes of multiple types of violence, but we helped lay the groundwork for those approaches to emerge.

VIOLENCE IS A LEARNED BEHAVIOR

I'd been anxious to connect with Dr. Deborah Prothrow-Stith since I'd seen her featured on *Frontline*,[9] where she voiced a new way of thinking about violence. I learned she was giving a talk at the University of California at Berkeley and went to hear her speak. Due to a bureaucratic mix-up, the talk was cancelled—a very lucky happenstance as it turned out, as we went to lunch instead.

Prothrow-Stith was among the very first to broadly reframe youth violence as a preventable public health crisis in the United States, catalyzing the modern movement to prevent street violence. As an extremely eloquent physician, she made the point that violence wasn't just a policing issue but that health and prevention could make important contributions to how we respond to violence.

On *Frontline*, Prothrow-Stith showed the curriculum she had designed for engaging youth, schools, and entire communities. The goal was to mobilize community resources and activate schools and local organizations around a core concept: nothing is to be gained by fighting. The curriculum itself was a valuable step forward. Just as important, I thought, was the notion the curriculum promoted—violence is a learned behavior, which can be unlearned, and different behaviors can be learned instead. Despite being located at opposite ends of the country, she and I resolved to integrate that thinking and approach with the coalition and movement I was trying to further in California.

In her nightly residency work in the emergency room at Boston City Hospital, Prothrow-Stith was increasingly saddened and frustrated as she encountered a steady stream of young Black victims of violence. She quickly discovered that in her role as medical provider, she wasn't expected to address the behavior of her patients or the community conditions or culture that made street violence more likely to occur. Emergency department doctors wouldn't release heart patients without prescriptions and referrals, nor would they release those who had attempted suicide until they were confident these people were not at risk of reattempting. Yet patients who'd been stabbed or shot due to community violence simply got stitched up and released, without concern for their state of mind or the environments they were going back to.

Since street violence was addressed only as a clinical issue, and family violence, child abuse, domestic abuse, and so forth were considered family issues, doctors and hospitals hadn't yet implemented interventions, such as universal screenings that ask about exposure to domestic violence. Likewise, patients had very little access to mental health services that can alleviate trauma and potentially prevent future incidents. These later developments in early identification have been critical both for the individual experiencing violence and potentially to learn about patterns of violence in communities—although even these interventions come after actual violence has occurred. Prothrow-Stith came to realize that violence was, in effect, a *chronic* issue; many of the patients she saw appeared in emergency rooms and had contact with the criminal justice system again and again as victims, witnesses, or perpetrators—often interchangeably. Spending billions suturing and incarcerating[10] people involved in and exposed to violence, year after year, without addressing the underlying concerns is both heartbreaking and futile.[11,12]

As much as anything, Prothrow-Stith brought compassion to her focus on violence affecting youth. She challenged the assumptions that lead to blame and incarceration: that violence is always an individual's choice, that punishment or the threat of it is both warranted and an effective deterrent, and that violence is an inevitable aspect of some people's behaviors. Prothrow-Stith shared with me that growing up in a faith-oriented Black community in the South, she didn't have the notion that violence was a natural or inevitable expression; instead, she believed dignity and respect were true Black norms. As she was treating her patients, she recognized that violence was too often expected from and imposed onto the culture of Black communities, which in itself undermined individuals' dignity and self-respect.

Prothrow-Stith knew it didn't have to be that way. In her book *Deadly Consequences*, she states, "Poor people do not choose to live in a battle zone, their lives constricted by tragedy and hopelessness. Poor teenagers are no different from other adolescents. [...] What separates armed teenagers in inner city neighborhoods from their more affluent peers are the choices that are available to them. [...] We can nourish them by providing them with better choices."[13]

Incorporating this understanding, Prothrow-Stith and another violence researcher, Dr. Howard Spivak, reached out to young men in the ER to support their healing and help them overcome trauma. Living in a violent environment had literally rewired their brains as a coping and survival mechanism. Prothrow-Stith and Spivak guided them in learning to manage anger and impulses while redeveloping empathy and problem-solving skills. They understood that friends and supportive family can play a significant role in reversing harmful behaviors, since most people engaged in violent acts know one another. Prothrow-Stith's Violence Prevention Project coined the phrase, "Friends for life. Friends don't let friends fight."[14] The idea is that friends should feel empowered to remind each other that fighting isn't needed, rather than making one another feel weak or less masculine for not fighting. Also, friends should know it's okay to respond to violence in nonviolent ways and not egg each other on during fights or incite violence for attention or power.

Over time, in addition to developing our local work, Prothrow-Stith and I continued to build our collaboration. She taught the first graduate public health course on community violence at Harvard, and I followed by teaching a similar course at the University of California at Berkeley. We realized that our joint efforts could be considered a national approach. With this in mind, we partnered to provide training on violence prevention across the country. Encountering growing interest in prevention in cities in virtually every state, we developed a leadership training model, funded by the federal government, and helped further the skills and thinking of several hundred emerging leaders nationally.

L.A. AS AN EPICENTER

I first met Billie Weiss as she was starting a coalition to prevent violence in Los Angeles. She had heard about the efforts of Contra Costa County's AVAC and wanted to know how the success working collaboratively could be applied to L.A., which had significantly high rates of violence. I saw great potential in the new coalition's leadership building upon our AVAC model, and I knew that if we could make an impact in L.A.—the largest population center of the largest state in the country—it would have state-wide and national implications that would carry a lot of political weight. Also, because L.A. is the primary production home of movies and TV shows, I hoped that as norms around violence in L.A. shifted, it might permeate the entertainment industry and influence the industry to take better responsibility for the way it glamorizes violence and shapes so much of our culture. Also, since the same local newspapers and media outlets report on the coalition and on entertainment, articles about the coalition and its joint community work would be read by members of the industry.

Uniquely, Weiss came to this work by way of her career as a professional modern dancer. She understood performance, art, business, culture, and family—just the right skill set for launching a new endeavor in L.A. When she was ready for her life's Act II, she pursued her lifelong love of science, studying epidemiology—the study of the patterns, causes, and effects of health conditions—in order to help shape policies and practices to prevent illnesses. As a mother of five, she was particularly interested in children's health. To Weiss's astonishment she discovered that L.A. youth faced a far worse epidemic than any disease: violence. She learned that after year one of life, injuries and trauma exceeded disease as the leading cause of death of children and adolescents.[15] Over a thousand people were murdered in L.A. each year in the 1990s.[16] In fact, homicide has been the leading cause of death in the United States among young Black men between the ages of fifteen to twenty-four for more than ten years.[17]

In addition to movies and television programs heavily relying on violence and conflict for entertainment, positive news stories about young people are rare, and the news presents a cumulative picture that is distorted, conflating youth, race, crime, and violence. This creates a skewed view of who commits crime and who suffers from violence[18] and contributes to the view of violence as inevitable rather than preventable. Although youth were most likely to be the victims, terms like "youth violence" were generally understood to mean that youth were the problem, and they were treated more likely with fear than with sympathy—particularly Black and Latino children. In fact, the term "youth violence" seemed inextricably tied to race. According to my colleagues Lori Dorfman and Larry Wallack, who study the impact of media coverage of violence, "The result is a misinformed public motivated by fear to be more accepting of punishment-oriented public policies that are often discriminatory"[19] and are thus less likely to accept policies that effectively prevent violence. As well as working to change norms around violence and the frame in the media, we are careful in all of our work to say "violence affecting youth" so as not to stigmatize youth.

Weiss's new bosses at the health department liked her idea for creating a violence prevention initiative but didn't fund it. Pretty much no county did—most localities paid for public health and health services through state or national funding (in addition to receiving payments for treatment and direct services). There was almost no state or federal funding specifically for violence prevention, so, given the limited local resources, they had never worked on violence, even though it was a major cause of death and disability. Besides, preventing violence seemed like too much of a stretch and not their turf—they had the viewpoint, common in the medical and health arena, that attention to diseases is more important than injuries. Even the Centers for Disease Control and Prevention didn't establish a violence prevention center until 1994.

However, Weiss made the point that street violence was not a standalone problem. The most affected communities were facing poverty, discrimination, and unemployment, which also lead to other physical and mental health challenges and diseases. In communities with pervasive violence or where residents have fear of violence, people are less likely to walk and talk on the streets, parents don't allow their children to play or bike outside or walk to school, businesses are less likely to open and invest in neighborhoods, and there is less investment in improving deteriorating parks, housing, and schools.[20] Reduced options for healthy eating and activity exacerbate already existing illnesses and increase the risk for illness to develop.[21]

To succeed, the coalition had to be comprehensive, cross-cutting, and norms-changing. I suggested to Weiss that she identify collaborators using the broadest possible definition for violence prevention work. I have always found that people concerned about preventing violence come from different walks of life, with a capacity to contribute unique, complementary skills and perspectives. So Weiss organized a diverse group: community members, service providers, educators, artists, business people, ministers, youth, law enforcement, and health providers, setting the stage for the development of the Violence Prevention Coalition of Greater Los Angeles. The Coalition served as a concrete "hub" for violence prevention, building capacity, fostering dialog, and providing training and shared learning. It brought together many individuals and strategies into a coherent whole, fostering an engaged constituency that cares about the issue, responds rapidly to calls for action, and knows they can rely on each other for support in their work. Over the next few years, the diversity of leaders that helped make L.A. safer was extremely impressive and remarkably effective.

It also became a forum for integrating the prevention approach with law enforcement. Also, because law enforcement is both a Los Angeles City and County function but public health sits only at the county level, this collaboration fostered critically needed conversation and relationships. L.A. was one of the first places in the country where law enforcement leaders formed the conviction and then stated clearly they couldn't solve the violence problem alone and, in fact, welcomed the complementary approach of community prevention. As Gil Garcetti, the city's former district attorney, says, "Spending our tax dollars on actually preventing crimes, instead of pursuing death sentences after they've already been committed, will assure us we will have fewer victims."[22]

The Coalition ensured that community members, including survivors of violence and those who were formerly incarcerated, play a crucial part in the work. "Nothing," Weiss says, "is more powerful than a mother who has lost a child to violence." Survivors include both those who were spared death, though they may have been seriously injured, as well as families and loved ones of the dead and injured, themselves scarred by the event or by ongoing exposure. For those who have been repeatedly involved in violence, often as perpetrator, witness, and recipient, working together and with advocates in a movement to change systems and prevent violence both helps anchor their own experiences and healing, rekindling empathy for themselves and others whom they may have lost due to repeated trauma, and helps shift other people's perceptions about violence.

We've heard repeatedly that when one is a survivor, that becomes one's identity and overshadows previous notions, assumptions, and even politics. Historically, victims and survivors of individual acts of violence, particularly those in more affluent communities, were often engaged in support of law enforcement and punishment solutions. However, working with the Coalition helped shift many survivors' understanding of what was truly needed to stop violence. For example, Charles and Mary Leigh Blek, white, wealthy Republicans from Orange County whose son was killed in a robbery, might not previously have been as aware of the impact of violence in other communities, particularly communities of color; but following the death of their son, they worked tirelessly to reduce violence and particularly as advocates for stronger gun regulations.

Father Greg Boyle, a member of the L.A. coalition, says, "Nothing stops a bullet like a job."[23] Knowing that a lack of educational and economic opportunities and a "lethal absence of hope,"[24] are key underlying factors contributing to desperation and violence, Father Greg started Homeboy Industries more than twenty-five years ago to help provide valuable job skills, income, and a positive sense of accomplishment to young people, many of them formerly incarcerated or gang-involved. They work together to run a café, catering business, grocery store, and farmers' markets. I eat at Homegirl Café whenever I go to L.A.—in addition to the critical work they're doing, they have the most delicious breakfasts. Local art is displayed throughout the restaurant. In addition to job training, participants receive trauma-informed therapeutic services and address anger management, relationship-building, parenting, mental health, substance abuse, and domestic violence. Importantly, participants find kinship, caring mentors, and hope.

According to Father Greg, it's never too late to repair this attachment and gain some resilience. He says, "Homeboy Industries has been the tipping point in changing the metaphors around gangs. We've engaged the imagination of 120,000 gang members and helped them to envision an exit ramp off the 'freeway' of violence, addiction, and incarceration."[25] Homeboy Industries is recognized as an international model. It's critical that we learn from and build on successful models like this as we address violence across the country.

Reverend Romey Lillie brought the Carter Center's Not Even One program to his congregation in Compton. It was created by ministers and public health advocates. Reverend Fred Smith, who created the name along with Reverend Gary Gunderson explains, "Maybe public health workers can be satisfied with a statistical goal like a 50 percent reduction in homicide; that would be impressive and valuable. But when we are ministering to our communities, our goal must be 'Not Even One.'"[26] Part of their process involves reviewing every child and teen death in their congregation to understand the circumstances. They ask the crucial question: What can we do differently so this doesn't happen again? For example, an eleven-year-old was killed in the street near his home an hour after school ended. The congregation realized that there weren't safe places for children to go after school, so they worked together to create more after-school and weekend youth programming. Not Even One is a statement of vision and faith. It's not to say we can stop every violent act now, but it's an aspiration and a pledge to do so.

Community members have also worked creatively to improve the overall community fabric in the L.A. neighborhood Boyle Heights. The neighborhood's safe open space—limited to freeway on/off ramps and a cemetery—had for years hampered neighbors' efforts to exercise, socialize, and access services locally. With the help of the Latino Urban Forum, residents united diverse members of neighborhood, business, and civic groups to leverage local government support for transforming a cracked sidewalk surrounding the Evergreen Cemetery into a one-and-a-half mile rubberized jogging path. Within six months, 1,000 community members were using it daily to walk, jog, and socialize. James Rojas, cofounder of the Latino Urban Forum, worked tirelessly to create the path. He says, "It gives the residents a stronger sense of identity and a real sense of pride. . . . The rate of violence—I won't say it's disappeared, but I think it's really gone down because people have a lot more ownership."[27]

Promoting nonviolence through public art has played an important part symbolically and practically. Participating in arts and other creative activities helps reduce children's engagement in violence. Murals and community art projects also help transform neighborhoods, reducing blight and building community harmony. The Violence Prevention Coalition of Greater L.A. hands out annual Angel of Peace Awards created by a sculptor friend of Billie Weiss's who melts down used firearms that were acquired through a Mother's Day gun buy-back program and shapes them into angels in recognition of community leadership in preventing violence. The artist also creates monumental sculptures (and has placed one near Ground Zero in New York) to symbolize peace. Transforming weapons into statues has historical significance: during the war of independence, US patriots who were fighting British rule tore down the statue of England's King George III and melted it into bullets, which they used against the king's troops.[28] Today's peace angels complete this circle, reminding us we need reconciliation, not war, to strengthen our families and communities.

The Coalition has significantly influenced the way violence is understood and addressed in L.A. (and across the country). It is a hub for bridging government- and street-level efforts as well as coordinating and elevating advocacy and policy efforts such as criminal justice reform and bans on gun sales and shows. The L.A. coalition measures its success by the increasing numbers of kids enrolled in community programs; by the rapidly growing network of organizations working on the issue; by city, county, and statewide policies; and, most important, by the dramatic reduction in violence. Billie credits the collaborative approach of coalition work with this reduction. She adds, "Nothing else really matters if we can't save our own children and keep them safe."[29]

A NEW YEAR'S DAY

I got a call very early on New Year's Day when I lived in New York's Upper West Side neighborhood. An acquaintance—someone who'd been at my apartment the night before for a New Year's Eve party—had been sexually assaulted and killed on her way home from my house. When the police contacted me, they said

*the details were too grisly to report publicly—even in hard-edged[ ]
and were being withheld to avoid creating citywide panic. Three [
officer called to say they'd found the killer, her ex-boyfriend. "Just a
relationship," he said. I heard the relief in his voice.*

Knowing it was intimate partner violence, he could make sense of it and dismiss it as an isolated incident that wasn't of larger concern. To me, the murder was unfathomable, and so was his relief. Every day 1,300 women in the United States are attacked in domestic violence disputes and hundreds more are sexually assaulted. Every 9 seconds a woman is assaulted or beaten.[30] One in every five undergraduate women experiences attempted or completed sexual assault.[31] One in three women has experienced violence from an intimate partner, and domestic violence accounts for a fifth of all violent crimes.[32] This is even more of a threat for people of color and people with low incomes, who make up a disproportionate amount of domestic violence survivors.[33]

Unlike with street violence, violence within the family rarely leads to calls to the mayor or city council to provide the solution. Rather, and too often, it's considered a private matter, and the question of blame is ignored, as if nothing can be done. This acceptance of violence within the home as a private matter both shames and silences people who experience violence and impedes those who would otherwise speak out against it. It also makes it harder to bring the violence into the policy arena. While a mayor's job can literally be at stake when people feel unprotected and at risk in their communities, elected officials don't feel as compelled to find solutions for violence that occurs behind closed doors.

The notion of violence as a private matter was one of five norms described by Prevention Institute that underlay the neglect and perpetuation of violence. Two of the other norms relate to traditional gender roles: a narrow definition of manhood and limited roles for women, who from a young age are often encouraged, through both subtle and overt messages, to act and be treated as objects by men. These build on norms related to power, where value is placed on claiming and maintaining control over others, which was also described by many in the feminist movement who saw the fundamental issue as one of oppression. The final norm is violence as the way we solve problems, where aggression is tolerated and accepted as normal behavior and can be used as a way to get what one wants.[34] (And it's a surprisingly large shift for many to consider that violence isn't normal behavior or a necessary way to solve problems.) We saw these norms play out in policies and laws; media, including news, entertainment, and advertising; workplaces and schools; and day-to-day interactions across communities. We thought an important part of the solution was to explicitly describe these norms and bring them to light—and to make the point that these patterns could be changed.

Although these norms were originally described as reinforcing domestic violence against women by men, it's critical to recognize that they apply to violence within nonheterosexual relationships as well. Further, as these norms prescribe traditional notions of masculine and feminine socialization, they also lead to violence against people who are transgender, lesbian, and gay, and the cultural norms that ignore and stigmatize these populations can also lead to further silence and perpetuation of violence.

Early on in the movement to address violence within the home, advocates focused on basic protections, such as the availability of shelters, so women had somewhere to go where they could live without fear or if they didn't have the means to leave a dangerous situation and live on their own. The focus expanded to the legal and criminal justice system, helping to develop laws to protect individuals from further violence. Advocates then engaged healthcare providers in developing practices for asking about violence in the home, both to emphasize the importance of talking about violence and to provide resources and support to those who were experiencing it. Groups like the Violence Prevention Coalition of Greater Los Angeles insisted that law enforcement and other institutions take these issues more seriously, advocating for clearing the backlog of rape kits and assuring that hospitals continue to participate in the collection of evidence to assist the prosecution of sexual violence.

These were needed and effective interventions. A focus on prevention and norms and policy change is also necessary to systematically change the underlying causes of violence. Such was the approach of the organization Futures Without Violence, founded more than thirty years ago by Esta Soler and today the most powerful and effective organization dealing with how norms interplay with violence. Futures Without Violence overtly confronts hidden violence within families and among friends and has continually questioned the norm that what goes on behind closed doors is nobody's business.

As I was first getting to know Soler, a new football team was founded in Oakland to replace the outgoing Raiders, who briefly relocated to Los Angeles between 1982 and 1994. The new Oakland Invaders sought to announce their arrival by posting a series of provocative billboard and bus ads across Oakland, ones that announced, "Listen. Or we'll break your face."[35] Violence in Oakland was particularly rampant then, and the team presumably sought to take up the city's problem as a marketing ploy. Soler confronted the team's owner, explaining that those ads influence how people think and behave.[36] At first the owner dismissed it as the advertising company's decision, but later, and to his credit, he eventually acknowledged that as the owner he had responsibility for the ads' messaging. He then paid for a series of high-profile ads deglamorizing violence and ran them on virtually every bus. He hosted events at the stadium, where players spoke out against violence toward women.

Soler has sought to address the norms, policies, and social systems that capitalize on unhealthy relationships. Ads, news reports, and movies often sexualize women while tacitly glamorizing violence against women. Women are still subject to significant inequities in hiring and pay (and even more so for women of color). Women encounter legal barriers to divorce, even in abusive relationships, and still face heavy stigma if they go public about being beaten, as though it were their fault.

Most important, Soler has elevated these issues in the national forum, playing a pivotal role in creating the Violence Against Women Act (VAWA) of 1994, the United States' first comprehensive federal legislation to end violence against women and children. The passage of the law was a statement that violence against women was not a private matter. And by defining how the criminal justice system should respond and improve services for victims, VAWA dramatically changed the nature and the seriousness with which violence against women was addressed, making it clear that the "power over" norm was unacceptable. In its first reauthorization, VAWA added housing rights, which was very important because women with housing alternatives are more likely to leave when domestic abuse is threatened. VAWA has since been reauthorized and expanded three times.

Recognizing that women of color, immigrants, native communities, and the LGBTQ population are at higher risk and were excluded from previous bills, reauthorizations have explicitly included those populations as well as prohibited LGBTQ victims from being turned away for services or protections based on sexual orientation or gender identity.

GUNS KILL PEOPLE

There are between 270 million and 310 million guns in the United States,[37] which equates to at least one gun per person. The United States has about twice the gun ownership per capita of the country with the next highest rate and at least four times the rate of every other country in the world. Research shows that access to firearms and other weapons greatly increases the risk of violence[38] and the availability of guns and ammunition greatly increases the likelihood of severe injury and death.[39,40] Most suicides and two-thirds of all homicides in the United States are gun-related,[41] and more than four out of five murdered children are killed with a firearm. More than a fifth of US teenagers report having witnessed a shooting.[42] Virtually all other countries look at the United States in disbelief: How could we do this to our families and communities? Why would we allow such risks? Getting rid of guns is not a moral issue. It's not even the goal—it's simply an effective method for saving lives. Guns don't just pose risks; they bring statistically certain outcomes.

In our ongoing onslaught of mass shootings, US legislators are afraid to tackle gun laws, even though the public overwhelmingly supports them. As Billie Weiss says, "Firearms are the new F-word." Following the close presidential election of 2000, the National Rifle Association (NRA) took credit as the deciding element, promulgating the notion that Al Gore's pro-gun–control stance cost him the presidency.[43] The NRA pledged to oppose—and defeat—all politicians who dared to speak up for sensible gun laws. They effectively interspersed gun rights into the US conservative agenda, making it a litmus test like abortion.

Even the Centers for Disease Control and Prevention (CDC) was effectively bullied into not studying gun deaths by the NRA: CDC funding contracts specifically state that parties receiving CDC funding may not advocate or promote gun control,[44] including several initiatives on which my organization took the lead.[45] This has been construed to include restrictions on any research in gun-related outcomes. Former Arkansas Rep. Jay Dickey,[46] who sponsored the original bill restricting gun research, now says the restrictions have gone too far and that he wants Congress to repeal the limits on gun research.[47] These efforts continued to build, and in 2008 the currently conservative Supreme Court for the first time interpreted the Second Amendment of the US Constitution as protecting an individual's right to have a gun, marking a significant shift in national policy. The decision found Washington, DC's Firearms Control Regulation Act to be unconstitutional—the law had been in place since 1975 and banned residents from owning handguns, automatic firearms, or high-capacity semiautomatic firearms, as well as prohibited possession of unregistered firearms.[48] As people across the country become fed up and alarmed that NRA mandates have shifted the national landscape and shaped policies, reversing or preventing most common-sense gun regulations,[49] solutions are emerging at local levels.

When the NRA and other efforts to interfere with gun restrictions began to build in the 1990s, I collaborated with a coworker, Andres Soto, to lodge a visible response. To start, we analyzed the list of registered gun dealers in Contra Costa County. What we found was vexing: hundreds of gun owners had acquired a misleading "dealer" designation but were in many cases simply residences where individuals sought more flexibility in purchasing and owning guns in a manner that shirked sales tax.

We translated this discovery into a form of "social math" to help make the information more relevant and understandable—showing that the number of gun dealers exceeded the number of fast-food restaurants and gas stations combined. We mapped their location in each city to bring the issue closer to home, which appealed to local news outlets. People were suddenly aware that they and their children lived near hidden gun caches. The project reinforced that gun availability wasn't just abstract; it was about children's safety.[50]

This created an enormous outcry. Even some people who owned guns themselves felt committed to regulating gun distribution in the community. However, preemption laws prevented us from passing laws restricting sales of guns in the county. So we developed a more creative strategy: gun dealers, like any business owners, had to maintain a business license, meet zoning requirements, and collect and pay sales tax. It turned out that very few of the dealers complied with any one of these laws, let alone all three.

The media swarmed. These findings meant that there were 462 gun dealers in the area that for the most part the government didn't know existed. As a result of this information campaign, the public learned that virtually all the gun dealers were out of compliance, and in nearly every case they voluntarily decided not to continue being dealers—the number of dealers dropped from several hundreds to a handful, making local communities and families more secure.

At the request of Contra Costa County's Board of Supervisors, we developed a countywide Action Plan for Violence—not only addressing guns but violence generally, especially street violence. It was the first comprehensive public health and prevention strategy in the country, and, to my surprise, the Board put this on the ballot along with two other advisory issues on bullets and assault rifles.

Hundreds of thousands of voting adults received the ballot arguments to read as part of their election packets. Combined with heavy press coverage, this prompted them to think about violence as a key community prevention issue and to consider three questions: Did they want a comprehensive approach to preventing violence? Did they want to pass a ban on assault rifles? And would they pass a new tax on bullets, which was a new strategy for reducing gun violence? All three initiatives passed with an overwhelming mandate, all passing with nearly two to one in favor. They passed in the low-income neighborhoods where violence was most prevalent and they passed in primarily higher income, mostly white neighborhoods as well. The success of these local initiatives sent strong messages to state and federal legislators that communities want stricter firearm regulations and a stronger focus on violence prevention. Strategies like this should be repeated now, so they will bubble up and spread, empowering more and more communities to keep their residents safe.

I was invited to testify at the National Science Foundation's Institute of Medicine about our work. Though I felt a bit intimidated on this national stage, building on my direct community experience and knowledge, I spoke with passion, empathy, and, I hoped, persuasion. The speaker who followed me was Wayne La Pierre, the recently appointed NRA CEO, who dismissed my testimony as unfounded rhetoric, saying that our commit-ment to community efforts was "naïve" and that our ballot initiatives were "meaningless." I was shocked at how disregarding and unrealistic his com-ments were. Regrettably, in that format I wasn't given a chance to respond. The third panelist, however, detailed everything I yearned to say.

Dr. Gary Slutkin was an epidemiologist who had spent a decade shap-ing World Health Organization strategy for fighting AIDS in Africa. He was returning to his home in Chicago, and, as he later told me over cof-fee, was convinced he could overcome violence there by applying similar strategies.

Slutkin developed Cure Violence, a foremost national and interna-tional initiative for interrupting violence. He calls it a norms-change pro-gram, and it's a powerful method of applying violence prevention strategy one person at a time and, subsequently, changing the expectations and behavior within a community. Cure Violence hires survivors, individuals who in many cases have been incarcerated and/or gang members, as the "experts" who know what's going on in the community and who know how to best intervene. It then trains them as outreach workers called violence interrupters. These advocates enact community mobilization to connect with at-risk youth to prevent violence and shootings by identifying and mediating potentially lethal conflicts, following up to ensure that the con-flict does not reignite, and changing beliefs about the acceptability and inevitability of violence. Since this model was created in Chicago, sixteen other cities, including L.A., have adopted it as a part of their violence pre-vention and intervention strategy. Overall, Cure Violence has measured a significant drop in shootings and killings and an almost 100 percent drop in retaliation murders.[51]

As disheartening as my encounter with Wayne La Pierre was, my ini-tial encounter with Slutkin, an ongoing colleague and friend, made the trip more than worth it.

TRAUMA IS MAKING US SICK

I was taking a break from work and reading about basketball on the Internet. I saw on the right of the screen an article about a young teen who killed his parents in their Oakland home. I clicked on it, and as I read, it started to filter into my consciousness that I knew them. We shared close friends and the mother had visited my home. The son and I had gone for a long walk with my dog, and he was very sweet and thoughtful. I didn't know the details of his history but understood that he had a very challenging and traumatizing early childhood. I remember that it had been called a high-risk adoption when my friends became his parents. Though they brought him needed compassion, safety, and support, clearly the impact of his profound trauma on his responses and behavior had not completely healed. In the end, he said that, knowing she would be angry that he skipped school and was home, he strangled his mother. Then he waited for his father to come home and did the same thing. Now both parents were dead and the son would soon be imprisoned for life. It was beyond-belief horror.

I remembered a Justice Department convening I had attended over fifteen years earlier for the first meeting of Safe from the Start, a program initiated by Janet Reno when she was the US Attorney General. I remember Eric Holder, then Deputy Attorney General and later US Attorney General in the Obama Administration, presenting a chart that showed a child, "Chris," with a history of criminal justice involvement—starting as a witness to spousal violence at age three and continuing to his sixtieth encounter with the system following his participation in a heinous act of violence. They made the point that earlier intervention was central to preventing later problems. Needless to say, witnessing violence is traumatizing, perhaps even more so at a young age. This child—then only sixteen—had had too many violent experiences and chronic trauma, without enough supportive responses to overcome the impact.

At about that time, Dr. Vince Felitti, whom I met later on, was taking a systematic look at how early exposure to violence and other trauma play out later in life. Working with Kaiser Permanente's vast database of long-term patients, Felitti found that what he called adverse childhood experiences (ACEs) accumulate and people who had experienced trauma when they were young—including being neglected, witnessing or experiencing violence, or living in a home with someone who had mental illness or addiction or who was incarcerated—were at greater risk of having serious health problems as they aged. Strikingly, ACEs are so destructive they increase the likelihood of developing virtually every other health problem, from anticipated ones such as depression, drug use, alcoholism, and other mental health challenges to illnesses such as asthma, heart disease, and diabetes. Exposure to trauma also leads to increased risky behavior for children, including early initiation of smoking, sexual activity, and pregnancy; antisocial attitudes; lack of involvement in activities and school; and poor academic performance.[52]

While most people who have experienced early trauma don't end up in the cycle of violence, it's still *far more likely* that they will.[53] As Felitti's work showed, children who experience trauma early in life are at greater risk for engaging in a variety of types of violence, including child and elder abuse, intimate partner violence, and suicide. It was also shown that survivors of one form of violence are more likely to be victims of other forms of violence, confirming AVAC's conclusions that violence is tied to early life events and that various forms of violence are interconnected—though AVAC had not named *trauma* as the critical link.

Caring adult intervention for a young person exposed to trauma strengthens resilience and acts as a protective factor. Our colleague Jim Garbarino pointed out at the time that having more resilience factors such as ongoing support and resources was "compensatory,"[54] reducing the likelihood that children will engage in violence and other high-risk behaviors and increasing the chances that they will have positive perspectives and behaviors, such as healthy eating, success in school, self-control, and healthy relationships.[55]

Later, I spoke with Felitti at a Department of Justice hearing in Detroit about the importance of his research, which I used to describe as some of the most significant *unrecognized* research on children's well-being. Then recently, due to many people's collective work to increase understanding about the community environment's impact on health and safety, a tipping point was reached and Felitti's research was brought to light—the health world embraced the role of ACEs in children's development. Dr. Felitti and I discussed this very positive shift to an intention of trauma-informed healthcare but also the need for moving beyond healthcare to changing the community environments that foster the violence and trauma in the first place.

Felitti's ACE studies happened over a generation ago,[56] and while it's certainly intuitive that personally experiencing violence can lead to trauma and health challenges, we are now learning that in many neighborhoods across the United States, entire communities experience traumatic events and chronically traumatizing conditions, which directly impact community members' physical and emotional health. The presence of chronic trauma also impacts service providers and first responders.

All people and communities deserve equal opportunities to be healthy and safe, but we know that these opportunities are not distributed evenly across US society. Experiencing or fearing violence in the street, in homes, and in relationships also causes trauma and has immediate and long-term emotional and mental health consequences, and this is more common in communities with deteriorated living conditions, poverty, racism, and lack of educational and economic opportunities. When children are in fear, they can't focus on learning, contributing to illiteracy, bullying, truancy, and high dropout rates. Trauma can become a basis for how people perceive and respond to events in their lives.

Alternatively, the presence of quality schools, health and mental health facilities, libraries, recreational centers, and parks buffers against the likelihood of violence and chronic trauma. Students of color are also more likely to be punished, expelled, or arrested for infractions while at school, which in turn reduces graduation rates and academic achievements[57] and increases the likelihood of involvement and exposure to violence. Students and their parents in predominantly white and affluent communities are provided more access to support systems and have disproportionately higher rates of academic success.[58] This difference in outcomes makes sense, but it's also completely preventable.

Engaging children in a love of learning and providing the resources for learning are also vital. The city of Salinas, for example, did a smart thing by partnering libraries with schools as one facet of its violence prevention strategy. Providing all students with free library cards, exempt from fines, prompted kids to read and use the library. This enriched children's experience and offered a safe alternative to the streets after school. The L.A. Unified School District is also attempting to shift the norms that lead to punishing children. The school board passed a policy banning defiance as grounds for suspension. The policy implemented support and incentives district-wide to promote positive behavior. Across the country, 13,000 schools are using this approach, which has reduced office discipline referrals by up to 50 percent, significantly improving children's opportunity to learn.[59]

We now know that, to support healthy communities, we have to anticipate and be systematically accountable for the elements that have led to high levels of violence and trauma and work to create resiliency in communities. As Howard Pinderhughes, expert on youth, race, and violence at the University of California at San Francisco, says, "There are places and spaces where hope exists, and positive work is going on in many communities. There are many organizations and people trying to create communities where everyone can thrive—young people, working people, people who are elderly, and the whole community. The most influential voices should be these institutions, norms, and individuals in a community who are engaging in that work. That is the goal and the vision for how you move beyond community trauma into a thriving community."[60]

UNITY

In 2005 the Prevention Institute partnered with the CDC on an initiative called UNITY, short for Urban Networks to Increase Thriving Youth through Violence Prevention. Borne of the recognition that urban areas carry many of the greatest burdens of chronic street violence—and, not coincidentally, the most poverty and racism—we aimed to apply a prevention model to violence in major American cities.

At the time UNITY was launched, it included many of the largest cities in the United States. Billie Weiss assessed their existing prevention efforts by sampling a third of the largest US cities. She found cities with the greatest success in preventing violence (and the lowest rates of violence) were the ones that employed the broadest collaboration, not those with a standout program or the strongest policing.[61] This was a significant finding, and it changed the way cities thought about prevention.

In short, it takes teams of people and communities focused on preventing violence pulling together to make a difference. In urban settings, where violence is likely to proliferate, collaboration involves ensuring that every government agency sees violence prevention as part of its job—and that each plays a key role in fulfilling it. Mayors participating in UNITY have combined resources from not just public health, law enforcement, and criminal justice but also art, education, housing, economic development, parks, and transportation, as well as faith leaders, business and community leaders, youth, and survivors.

When I first heard the term "cross-sector collaboration," while I was at an international safety conference in Sweden, I wasn't sure what the term meant or how it was much different from the coalitions with which I was already engaged. I soon realized that the Europeans were more explicit and deliberate in bringing together different sectors of government. Thus, it wasn't just like-minded groups saying, "How do we accomplish a goal together?" It was multiple fields, with a range and diversity of goals saying, "How do we creatively broaden our thinking and join forces, so we can accomplish the big, important work that government should achieve, which might otherwise go unnoticed?"

The active collaboration of multiple sectors—or in the case of government, agencies and departments—to account for the health and safety impacts of their decisions has been dubbed "health-in-all-policies." Adopting a health and safety-in-all-policies approach not only builds a health and safety viewpoint into strategies and decisions, but it also augments the agency-specific goals and responsibilities. For example, redevelopment projects would consider how to foster access to safe parks for physical activity and safe and easy access to public transit. Education initiatives would examine underlying issues affecting school attendance and performance, encourage solutions that don't criminalize some children while providing support to others, and also support safe-routes-to-school programs.

Through these city-level collaborations, Rachel Davis—who leads UNITY and all violence prevention efforts at Prevention Institute—captured the best practices for cities in the form of the UNITY Roadmap.[62] The roadmap emphasizes prevention as a multielement framework for assessing issues, assets, and priorities in a given municipality and again in designing comprehensive, sustainable solutions for violence that bring together proven, cross-cutting strategies in a coherent system.

Such strategies might include simultaneous efforts to invest in schools, create jobs, mentor youth, reduce alcohol density, and offer social services—all alongside strengthening existing law enforcement and the judicial process. These efforts build on one another, and, as they mature they can lead to (and even produce) peripheral gains: cleaning up parks, removing blight, supplying fresh foods, building public transportation systems, repairing housing, and greening public spaces. In other words, these strategies simultaneously reduce violence and improve health.

The city of Philadelphia demonstrated these principles when it started greening vacant lots to encourage private housing and business development in its underserved neighborhoods. As the Pennsylvania Horticultural Society rallied city agencies and community-based groups to remove debris from the lots and plant greenery, formerly incarcerated residents were trained and hired to maintain the spaces. A study evaluating this effort later found that greening the vacant lots and keeping public spaces clean was linked to fewer gun assaults and less vandalism.[63]

UNITY's nationwide results have been impressive. Rates of violence, including suicides, are down in almost every UNITY city—despite a national proliferation of guns, spike in suicides, and the economic downturn that have impacted at-risk youth and disenfranchised communities disproportionately. Many UNITY cities have increased their collaboration and deepened their understanding of why public health and prevention are crucial, and now most have turned their individual attentions to implementing additional short- and long-term strategies. This is all new. When we launched UNITY, most cities lacked comprehensive approaches. Now public health is playing a central role, advancing strategic plans, running coalitions, and engaging youth and other stakeholders in high-violence neighborhoods. It is helping leaders design system-wide solutions and leverage assets more effectively.

UNITY's architects have also learned that this work must be done in support of and in partnership with community members to build on their efforts and address their needs. When developing new initiatives, securing community involvement and leadership is critical to success, including community-based organizations, families, community members, former gang members, formerly incarcerated individuals, and survivors of violence. Supporting community members as leaders and encouraging collaboration among community partners early on builds trust and a common understanding and language, helps identify the most important local priorities and needs, builds on existing community strengths and values, and enhances buy-in from those who will be most affected by the strategies that are put in place.

Minneapolis, once nicknamed Murderopolis, became an early UNITY partner when Mayor J. T. Rybak saw the opportunity to tackle the underlying issues spurring violence. A team of city officials from multiple sectors and diverse community stakeholders led an eight-month collaborative design process, producing the Blueprint for Action: Preventing Youth Violence in Minneapolis.[64] Employing a comprehensive, public-health approach that involves community leadership at every level, the Blueprint's goals are to address the underlying contributors to violence and significantly reduce and prevent youth violence using a combination of public health and law enforcement strategies. The plan includes ensuring that all youth have connections to trusted adults, intervening with youth at the first sign of risk, bringing young people back from the brink, and helping create an environment where children unlearn a culture of violence.

"This approach works," says Minneapolis Police Department Lieutenant Michael Sullivan. "It's working right here, right now, in my city, where we reduced violence by 40 percent in just two years—and then brought it down another 20 percent. And we didn't do it by increasing arrests. We did it by giving young people opportunities to thrive."[65] As part of its blueprint, the city has funded more than a dozen community organizations to support youth employment, academic enrichment, and numerous other community-based solutions. Following this success, in 2009 the city expanded from a focus on five neighborhoods to the twenty-two neighborhoods most impacted by violence.

WE KNOW WHAT TO DO

As I was reviewing the conclusion to this chapter, I received the following note from a colleague (names and locations have been removed, but it could take place in any part of the United States): "I just wanted to reach out and let you know that Baby X was killed by a stray bullet from a gang shooting and died last night. Not only was the baby born at our medical center, but her mother participated in our Employment, Education, Case Management and Mentoring

Programs while pregnant. Mom is from a multigenerational gang family but made a significant effort to provide a better life for her baby. Gang violence doesn't get any worse than this. No words can describe the feelings I had today as I looked at the baby's blood still on the driveway concrete."

Whenever I hear about an incident like this, I feel sick and enraged because violence isn't inevitable. We know what to do to prevent violence in the United States right now, which gives me hope. Rates of homicides and serious assaults could be reduced by more than half if we put the effort and resources into their prevention. Less than a generation after we started treating violence as a preventable issue, we are already seeing significant success.[66] We've come a long way, but we haven't yet coalesced into one unified movement to prevent violence. It's time to bring successful efforts to scale. It's unconscionable if, as a nation, we don't.

Of course, we need to further refine and advance our knowledge of how to prevent violence, while we systematically implement what we already know works. Whenever I say this, people always ask, "What is it? What *is* this approach that works?" Well, it's not one thing. No single program can address the magnitude of the issues that come with violence or the diverse factors that cause it. It takes a deliberate allocation of resources and political will. It's about moving away from alcohol as a pastime, from incarceration as the answer, from violence as the norm and the solution, from marketing and media that glorify violence. It's about providing affordable housing, quality education, and living-wage jobs; investing in economic renewal for all neighborhoods; improving community living conditions; and ensuring safe streets and access to healthy foods—across the board.

It's unreasonable to blame certain individuals, families, communities, or schools for the exposures and behaviors that lead to violence. We must shift the still-prevailing notion that violence is about individual choice, about bad people doing bad things. The use and acceptance of incarceration of young people in the United States is far greater than in any other country.[67,68] Clearly this is the opposite of an investment in prevention. Despite the fact that the juvenile justice system was created with the belief in prevention and rehabilitation for children, currently its major responsibility is punishment, which hasn't been shown to be effective for preventing further violence. By the age of twenty-three, over a third of US youth (and half of young Black men) have been arrested.[69]

These numbers are unfathomable. There are tremendous inequities across the criminal justice system by race—more police stops, more arrests, and longer jail sentences for people of color. This means that for Black children the estimated likelihood that one of their parents will be imprisoned by the time they are fourteen years old is one in four.[70] (For white children, the likelihood is one in twenty-five.) Black people are imprisoned at nearly six times the rate of whites, and Latinos at nearly double the rates of whites,[71] even for similar offenses. In addition to being inhumane, it's also extraordinarily expensive. We could instead invest that money in decent schools, mental health and social services, parks, and communities.

Violence is frequently intergenerational, and we now understand the relationships between different types of violence. Because forms of violence are interconnected, reducing the presence of one type reduces others. It is time to advance the interrelated solutions that address all the underlying causes of violence. If we reduce trauma, shift norms, reduce the impact of alcohol and other drugs, and move instead to supporting families and communities, we will see less child abuse, intimate-partner violence and sexual assault, and street violence.

One key to reducing interrelated forms of violence is reducing trauma, at both the individual and at the community level. Acknowledging the cumulative impact of stressful experiences and risk factors in the environment is a crucial start; next we need to develop a comprehensive framework for preventing and healing community-level trauma. While we don't yet have this framework, our colleagues are laying the foundation. We're digging deep into the relationships between inequities, violence, and community trauma to understand the systematic effects of trauma at a community level and how community trauma undermines individual, family, and collective resiliency in the face of violence.[72]

Another element of reducing interrelated forms of violence is focusing on healthier norms. American culture promulgates violence in many ways. Unhealthy products that glorify and encourage violence are promoted—including guns, alcohol, and video games. Media also act as a megaphone, broadcasting violence as sexy, powerful, and normal. It's a profitable strategy for vested businesses, but at what cost? Norms change is doable, though at first it seems insurmountable. The misogyny that was rampant on sports talk, for example, has now become unacceptable, and we have seen suspensions and resignations over comments that a few years ago would have been accepted or ignored.

Alcohol use exacerbates every type of violence, and alcohol is involved in two-thirds of all homicides.[73] Alcohol ads often build on unhealthy traditional norms about men's and women's roles, promising male sexual dominance through drinking. Changing policies and practices surrounding alcohol sale is very successful in reducing violence across the board.[74] Incidents of violence have been dramatically lowered by curtailing sales of single-serving alcohol, instituting server intervention programs, contesting alcohol ads and sponsorships, and prohibiting alcohol sales at the end of sporting events.

Community Coalition—a nonprofit organization that works with Black and Latino residents to build a prosperous and healthy South Los Angeles—launched a grassroots advocacy campaign to use L.A. County's local zoning and land-use regulations to reduce the number of alcohol outlets in the community as well as influence policies for conditional-use permits. Through community leadership and organizing and effective use of policy change, it ultimately succeeded in shutting down nearly 200 liquor stores. As a result of the coalition's activities, the neighborhood saw a 27 percent reduction in violent and drug-related crime within a four-block radius of each closed liquor store.[75]

Ultimately, our prevention efforts become truly effective once they rally broad-based community participation and build critical mass. We need to broaden who is in leadership, empowering and allowing space for youth, survivors, people of color, and other community members to play a leading role in advocating for community changes that will create an environment of dignified living, health, and safety for everyone. As Makani Themba Nixon, a leader in health justice, says, "Efforts that engage community residents and give them a sense of their own power can make a real difference in their ability to solve problems as well as strengthen individual members' sense of community. Community-based efforts to change policy not only address problems through the policy changes they achieve but also aid communities in addressing the factors that put them at risk in the first place."[76]

In order to move away from violence in communities, violence in homes, and the cycle of incarceration, we must improve education and employment opportunities.[77] Otherwise, many don't have the means to earn a living wage—without access to education, job training, support services, and loans, people are more likely to suffer from chronic stress and may need to turn to other means to meet basic survival needs, including the drug economy and other illegal activities, increasing their likelihood of being arrested and continuing the cycle.[78] Living-wage jobs are empowering and support dignity. When Father Greg Boyle talks about repairing the effects of trauma, he says, "Twenty percent is being part of a healing community. The other 80 percent is having a job and a paycheck."[79]

It's also time to change hiring practices that discriminate against people whose circumstances have led to engagement in the criminal justice system. Durham, North Carolina, is just one city that has removed questions about prior convictions from job applications. In 2011, before the city took that step, only 2 percent of hires had criminal records. Under the new policy, that figure rose to 4.5 percent in 2012, 9.4 percent in 2013, and 15.5 percent in the first quarter of 2014. The practice has increased economic opportunity without any increase in workplace crime.

All of these practices strengthen the social fabric of neighborhoods, which needs to happen across communities. Residents need to be connected and supported and feel that they hold power to improve the safety and well-being of their families. All residents need to have a sense of belonging, dignity, and hope. The resources and capacity to do this already exist—it just requires shifting decision-making about community outcomes back to communities and shifting funds from incarceration to supporting individuals, families, and communities. I'm encouraged to see that when Minneapolis updated its Blueprint for reducing violence, which is primarily focused on street violence, it added goals aimed at nurturing family systems and fostering violence-free social environments, which the coalition discovered were high-priority, crucial elements. The city has gone even further, developing a youth violence prevention legislative agenda, calling for a statewide policy that defines youth violence as a public health issue.

Preventing violence is complex, but it is doable and absolutely necessary for communities, families, businesses, and individuals to thrive. It boils down to making smart, caring investments in people, in the places where they live, and in the opportunities that enable them and our society to flourish. It takes vision, passion, and strategy as well as the right infrastructure to bring this to scale. The current generation's learning about prevention of violence provides a critical opportunity for the next generation of leaders, who must take what we know and put it to use to shift the public understanding of violence, further political will, advance a comprehensive policy agenda, and ensure successful strategies become common practice.

Eleanor Roosevelt asked, "When will our consciences grow so tender that we will act to prevent human misery rather than avenge it?"[80] The time is now. Our goal as a country should be to create healthy, resilient individuals and communities that are safe and just. This takes working together and requires all of us—from elected officials and business owners to community members, advocates, and practitioners—speaking up and saying we can, *and will,* do something to stop violence. Howard Spivak, now chief of staff for the National Institute of Justice, says, "We can do this; we know what to do; it's not rocket science, and we have the resources. Now we just have to do it."

[9]

WHEN PEOPLE THRIVE, BUSINESS THRIVES

I SMOKE FOR SMELL

I made a special trip from California to meet with Alan Blum, a family physician in Long Island, and we spent a Saturday talking at his home. He had come into the public light in an unusual manner: walking back and forth along the long, wide sweep of the Metropolitan Museum of Art's steps, protesting Phillip Morris's sponsorship of the very popular and well-publicized art exhibit, Art from the Vatican. Why would a doctor do such a thing, when he could be getting paid to treat patients? Dr. Blum's walk, which lasted for thirty days, captured the country's attention and raised important national questions.[1]

It's easy to see why sponsorship was a good investment for Phillip Morris. It's also become a familiar, though reprehensible, practice for an institution like the Metropolitan to accept any and all wealthy sponsors. How could we allow this to happen? Why should we permit a company doing so much damage to our health to benefit from the publicity and credibility associated with the Vatican and the Metropolitan Museum? Did we really want to be praising Philip Morris executives and honoring their brand?

Blum was among the first in the medical profession to directly and publicly criticize the tobacco industry. It had only been a few years since some doctors had advertised cigarettes with health claims. The American Medical Association had finally issued a statement about the dangers of tobacco (nearly always one of the last to take a strong position for health), yet the government was still giving out free cigarettes to armed services personnel.[2] Blum's advocacy was not only important because he was challenging tobacco but also because he was calling into question its marketing practices and our almost blind acceptance of them. We sold out so easily, without thinking, exchanging our health for a corporate contribution and allowing harmful industries to flip the notion of guilt by association and encourage "innocence by association." The environmental movement equivalent is greenwashing, when marketers try to make businesses look responsive to the environment and, thus, socially acceptable, by actions that do not fundamentally change their damaging products and practices.

Blum showed me the slides from the talks he gave to medical groups. Tobacco ads associated cigarettes with everything healthy, desirable, and successful. Special ads were created to appeal to women and to Blacks. He made counter billboards that he displayed in his talks and ads. His had ironic humor that ridiculed and transformed the cigarette ads to portray a more accurate statement of tobacco outcomes. "I smoke for taste" was a noted ad at the time, which sported an attractive man taking a thoughtful, sexy puff. In response, Blum produced an ad of someone with a cigarette dangling from his nose, which said, "I smoke for smell."[3]He revised a Virginia Slims ad (widely praised by some for its feminist message, "You've come a long way baby"[4]) and created Virginia Killers.[5]

Blum used advertising on the back of bus benches as a cost-effective way to gain a lot of attention. Daring the cigarette companies to sue him, he hoped it would lead to even greater exposure (they never did). He insisted on paid advertisements only, so people would realize this was an important issue. Public service announcements would be dismissed, he believed, as a weak government goody-goody health message. It's hard to tell exactly what led from one thing to another, but perhaps the Blum ads were the inspiration for the hard-hitting Truth Campaign ads and the courageous (for state government) campaign pioneered in California, which showed the Marlboro man, years later, on life support.

FOR THE LOVE OF COMMERCE

I grew up working in my father's business. He was a man who'd had to quit college after a year, abandoning his career aspirations to be a doctor to become a factory worker. He worked for his sister's husband, who I can say now—a family secret that's no longer necessary to keep, since all the principals have died—was a highly unpleasant man. So when my father returned to the factory after World War II, he saved the little he could for eight hard years and opened his own small fur factory, making mink coats and fur collars, which had just come into fashion.

At age ten, I started working Saturdays and school vacations; my older brother was doing so as well. The work was very hard, and it was incredibly hot and humid with the fur flying. I was constantly sweeping the showroom to literally "keep the fur down." I wasn't skilled at any of the labor, so I did the more basic tasks: removing the nails that stretched the furs, sizing the collars precisely, and delivering them to the coat manufacturers in the garment district. Since I was always good at math, I helped pay the bills and maintain the books. In that way, I started to appreciate how much hard work it takes to run a viable business.

The back and forth of negotiations intrigued me—the skill of deal-making, the decisions about pricing and risks, and the returns on wise choices. I learned that because the cost of the furs fluctuated wildly and we purchased them on credit before "the season," their worth, our potential profit, and the fashion trends themselves were all a big gamble. I began to understand the elements involved in making money and the savvy it took to be successful in business. In my father's case, profit margins were small, and he always needed to excel to stay ahead of the competition. His experience as an exploited worker made him a strong union supporter, and his values influenced me deeply. He encouraged his employees to take initiative and treated them well, believing that respect, fairness, and resourcefulness also enhance productivity and effectiveness. Viewing his business success as the result, in part, of their efforts, he took satisfaction in creating meaningful jobs. Some fellow business owners disagreed with his approach, but he proudly insisted it reflected core US work values.

LUNCH WITH THE GOVERNOR AND THE COKE REPRESENTATIVE

Business is the pulse of our country. We want commerce to be robust, because healthy communities and prosperity are natural allies. Many, if not most, businesses are fulfilling important community needs and wants, providing jobs, and encouraging productivity. When living-wage jobs are more plentiful and secure, people are better able to take care of their personal and family needs. They buy clothing, fresh food, and household goods; they are more likely to have adequate healthcare coverage; and they go out more, enjoying movies, restaurants, and culture. Stable employment and spending capacity buoy the economy, increasing personal and business prosperity in a mutually sustaining way.

Still, some businesses have spurned the community's needs by promoting health-damaging products, low wages, and poor working conditions. Large corporations, in particular, have been structured to make profit the primary value, overriding concerns for health and environment. As Marion Nestle, author of *Food Politics*, reminds us, the legal goal of corporations is not to achieve positive or healthful outcomes. Publically traded corporations are required, *by law*, to maximize profits for shareholders at all costs.[6]

In the midst of this pursuit, community conditions that foster health and safety often incur collateral damage. While this impact affects everyone, it harms populations that have become disenfranchised even more so. That's when the emphasis on profit tips out of balance, turning an asset into a detriment; in many cases, protective regulations are required to restore balance. When the *Wall Street Journal* reports, "The obesity problem is just a side effect of something good for the economy,"[7] we know we're paying too heavy a price for corporate profit-making.

While evaluating products and practices and addressing areas of concern, it's important to reemphasize the natural opportunity for synergy between commerce and communities. New opportunities are emerging for businesses to meet the consumer demand for health and wellness, just as the need to address climate change has stimulated energy innovation. Businesses fall along a continuum in terms of their contributions to personal and environmental well-being, and by developing products and practices that directly encourage health or clean energy, for example, companies can make a stronger contribution. Sound labor and manufacturing practices, the opportunity for workers to learn new skills, and workplace wellness policies are also immensely important contributions to health that businesses can make. Just as industry needs to acknowledge that a healthy workforce ensures its bottom line—and that healthy communities, including healthy customers, are essential—health advocates need to appreciate that business can contribute to well-being. The overarching narrative still holds true: business and good health align naturally, so consumer demand and national policies should protect and advance both together.

I was invited to a small group lunch with then-Governor Schwarzenegger to discuss strategies for improving healthy eating and physical activity. Our diverse group was aligned on many issues, but the rub came when we talked about soda. My colleague Harold Goldstein brought in pitchers of sugar to demonstrate the average US child's annual consumption from drinking sugar-sweetened beverages. A Coke representative, another invitee, first tried to divert the conversation by vaunting its contributions to the local community and then replied that soda itself is not a bad food; like any food, it can be over-consumed. "Overconsumed!" I thought. "That's a brilliant turn of words if you want to blame the customer." The evolution from a weekly soda-fountain treat to a multiple-soda-a-day habit didn't develop on its own. Drinking Coke has become a celebrated social norm, the result of a well-constructed, heavily funded marketing campaign: Coke is it—the REAL THING that helps drive the US epidemics in diabetes, heart disease, and stroke.

When products like cigarettes and soda harm our health, all organizations and industries wind up paying more for the resulting increase in healthcare costs, absenteeism, and lost productivity. It's time to remind businesses of this impact, encouraging them to align with health-enhancing efforts and to step up as advocates and core contributors to community wellness. Health advocates and consumers also need to be more sophisticated, challenging unhealthy businesses, supporting health-sustaining ones, and promoting the value of health for business success.

Increasingly soda is regarded as the new tobacco by those in the public health field: a heavily marketed product imposing enormous damage to the health of the populace and with little redeeming value as a producer. This wasn't widely understood when Governor Schwarzenegger became one of the first high-level politicians, and the first significant Republican, to take on the soda industry, which was then seen as an untouchable part of the more well-respected food industry. Of course, soda isn't the only very unhealthy food, but it is a good place to start fostering momentum for norms change because it is so heavily marketed, it has virtually no nutritional value, and there is a solid research base on its impact. The governor's initiative helped turn the tide, so California residents and others across the country understood it as an outlier. They could generally like business but question the soda industry. Our advocacy at that meeting—along with the governor's commitment to engendering health for California's youth and reducing risks of chronic disease—resulted in the elimination of soda and junk food in school lunches and vending machines;[8] ensuring fresh, free drinking water in every school; and strengthening physical activity standards.

SEVENTEEN

My uncle was the first marketing director of Seventeen *magazine, and he came up with the notion, back in the 1950s, that one could market to teenagers. I'm sure there were others who did that, but* Seventeen *was the first prominent teen magazine to identify children, girls in particular, as a market and as drivers of the economy. As a boy, I was fascinated by the allure of seventeen-year-old girls. I took it for granted that the magazine reflected their universal desires, never considering that different girls had different styles or tastes:* Seventeen *was authoritative.*

Seventeen dealt with fashion, makeup, and other things teenage girls might buy, like jeans. My uncle fully understood that a magazine called Seventeen *was equally aimed at thirteen-year-olds and that marketing to this age group could be very, very powerful. Of course, the whole point was to sell products and to capture the next generation of purchasers. Even then, marketers knew sex and beauty were top sellers, as they planted the early seeds of sexualizing women in advertising. My uncle had his own preteen daughter, and I wonder if he might have been concerned about his impact on girls like her. Instead, he probably valued her as a live-in example, where she could help refine his theories. Portraying kids as sexy was suddenly legitimized and celebrated as a part of progress—rather than being seen as pornographic. If it increased sales, it had to be good.*

My uncle also discovered, with the emphasis on youth culture and parents wanting to be ever-young, that teenagers could influence their parents' fashion choices and spending. This was especially true for women, and it turned out to be a major factor in Seventeen's *success. More than anything,* Seventeen *helped create teen shoppers, a market that was more than willing to see consumerism as a fulfilling way to live. Shopping became the reflection of one's persona and an emotional panacea.*

My uncle was well meaning and seemed very creative, but he didn't ask the fundamental questions: Do we want marketing and purchasing to be a major emphasis for our kids? Do we want to market our girls as sex objects? Do we want to allow advertising to twist social norms for the sake of making a profit at all costs? The early market just took these things for granted, admiring the innovation and my uncle as a genius—and he always enjoyed his renown and the money he earned from his prominence.

The late 1960s were a respite from the myths of the 1950s. Youth rebellion scrutinized everything from war to corporate abuses and our consumer culture. Burned bras and torn jeans made a strong statement that convention was neither favorable nor necessary—but then torn jeans became the fashion. Ironically, the whole counterculture became another excuse to pump up marketing, consumption, and profit. Ads picked up on this, setting the new images that would drive sales, and everything became a potential marketing device. Andy Warhol emphasized this by portraying Campbell's Soup as art and had the last laugh (all the way to the bank), with the soup can epitomizing contemporary art.

THE CONSEQUENCE OF STUFF

I remember my mother and father arguing; we had a 1950 Dodge that would never stop working, but my mother wanted something more glamorous. One day the car had a flat tire on the highway, and she had the junk man tow it away. My father bought it back for double the $50 she had been given, but three months later, he relented and we had a new car. I had loved the Dodge's long, racy fins that extended its back fenders and was sad to see it go.

One of the first big business practice scandals I can recall was "planned obsolescence," the idea that large corporations constructed their products, most notably cars, so they wouldn't last. The quality was intentionally limited, not maximized, so that repeat sales wouldn't dry up. Industry also figured out how to get people to replace their previously well-built products by creating an avid consumer culture, where new designs were *more fashionable* and people continually wanted the *next new thing*.

At first, this scandal, the first visible erosion of quality as an industry value, was not met with much shock. As Ronald Reagan crooned about "progress" and my father moaned about his Dodge, the suburbs seduced many, with their shopping malls and the ease and privacy of commuting in the latest model cars. Malls became the mecca for fulfilling the new consumer mantra—*more stuff now*. Of course, the suburbs were mainly for the *prototypical* "American" white, middle-class, upwardly mobile heterosexual families; TV could give all others the feeling that they were unimportant and left behind, and both subtle and overt policies ensured that suburbs, for the most part, stayed white.

Mall culture, along with the rest of suburban growth, brought its own health hazards, as buildings replaced green space and fast-food monopolies moved in. As traffic and populations increased, so did the potential for stress, asthma, and cancer. Chain and big-box stores blighted the horizon, stripping communities of their personal charm, local ownership, and business ingenuity. Consumers and manufacturers became partners in a way of doing business that was clearly starting to jeopardize people's health, safety, and mental well-being.

Further, suburbia itself became ground zero for one of the worst health concerns, the invisible chemical invasion. Chemicals could produce amazing results, and not many people worried about their "side" effects. These appealing, profit-enhancing outliers quietly infiltrated every product imaginable. In her iconic book, *Silent Spring*, environmentalist Rachel Carson wrote: "Kitchen shelf paper . . . may be impregnated with insecticide. . . . With push-button ease, one may send a fog of dieldrin into the most inaccessible nooks and crannies of cabinets, corners, and baseboards."[9] Carson portrayed wildlife dying and people contracting various diseases from the indiscriminate use of these "biocides." Ironically, the search for convenience inflicted ill health on the well-heeled, but, needless to say, low-income communities suffered the most egregious health impacts, as the predictable site of heavy industry and its toxic dumping. As a result of Carson's writing, environmental concerns became a national issue for everyday people.

People began to understand that the corporate agenda was becoming invasive and called for strategies aimed at recovering community values, health, and local culture. Planned obsolescence was the tipping point, where marketing things for profit as a business ethos trumped concern for workers, consumers, and health. Now we're in the consequence period, and it's not by accident. Industry's toxic residue has left communities— mostly disadvantaged ones—suffering from explosive rates of cancer, lead poisoning, and birth defects. Long-distance transportation of goods, including food, has caused stress, asthma, and cancer as well as excess greenhouse gases, resulting in long-term climate change and its related health and environmental impacts. Health effects from industry activity often manifest later, masking their connection and allowing corporations to dodge out. Work-related injuries, like mine collapses, have visible causes; increased rates of cancer and asthma resulting from multiple toxic sources are more complex to trace.

In her landmark book, *The Story of Stuff*, Annie Leonard reflects on our country's fascination with products, saying, "We've allowed our citizen self to be dwarfed by a relatively new reflex action—consume, consume, consume."[10] In exchange for constant replenishment of cheap things, the US consumer has condoned exporting jobs and manufacturing to countries where companies don't have to pay living wages, adhere to regulations, offer healthcare, or provide safe working environments. The US workforce has also suffered the ill effects of overseas competition, including a lack of living-wage jobs. Love of things cheap has also helped promote sugary drinks. A Berkeley colleague sent me photos of McDonald's ads for banned supersized drinks that were not only still being sold but were also discounted from 89 cents to 69 cents—so why have one soda a day when you can afford many? Featured on the sides of city buses, the ads are in Chinese, Vietnamese, and Spanish, clearly directed at populations who already suffer disproportionately from chronic diseases.

An overemphasis on stuff has also led to newer derivative products, such as payday loans. Many hard-working people must use payday loans to cover critical monthly expenses and emergency needs. Strapped borrowers keep rolling over loans in a vicious cycle of fees that's nearly impossible to escape. About $4.1 billion is spent annually on payday loan fees in the 32 states states that allow triple-digit interest rates.[11] Advocacy groups have succeeded in helping to pass legislation that outlawed triple-digit interest rates in eighteen states and the District of Columbia. Mike Donovan, former district director of operations for Check 'n Go, the country's second largest provider of payday loans, and the largest payday lender in Washington, D.C., became an advocate against the payday load industry and helped pass interest rate caps. Donavan said, "Of course, we train our sales staff to keep customers dependent, to make sure they keep re-borrowing, whether in the form of a renewal, or a back-to-back transaction, forever, if possible. We virtually guarantee customer retention by encouraging customers to borrow up to 85% of their gross income—that is, more money then they actually receive in their take-home pay. In Virginia, our policy is to loan 100% of gross income. . . . Let's talk about the industry's assertion that it does not target minority populations. I can tell you emphatically that it does. . . . We seek out low-income African American and Latino neighborhoods because we know that this is where our most profitable client base is located."[12] Rampant profiteering has ravaged health even more so in communities that have been disenfranchised, causing anger, frustration, and hopelessness to deepen.

WHEN WIN-WIN WON'T WORK

Before wrapping up the meeting, Governor Schwarzenegger turned the conversation away from soda's role in fostering chronic diseases, reminiscing about his personal experiences with Coke's sponsorships, as though Coke were a stodgy old friend, who may be politically incorrect but has a good heart. It was based on the "favors" Coke did for his mother-in-law, not coincidentally one of the Kennedys, in helping support the Special Olympics. And the Coke executive tried to use this friendliness to emphasize the goal of creating a win-win compromise. Perhaps, he suggested, we could all agree on focusing on physical activity instead of soda. But there was no consensus or basis for compromise, and Coke was neither a good friend nor a good business, if "good" means supporting people's well-being and not just corporate profit. We remained a group of health advocates facing a corporation charged with maximizing profit, regardless of—and here in opposition to—health. In fact, such antihealth corporations insinuate themselves into our lives and culture, equating their brands with our enjoyment and the good life—while giving all businesses a bad name.[13,14]

Win-win? Politicians may prefer it to taking sides between certain businesses and health, but it's a trap. Win-win doesn't actually work when one player is selling—and profiting highly from—poor health and is unwilling to make substantive changes to its products or practices. After all, why should advocates relent in defending well-being or allow unhealthy products to become the default marketplace options?

Businesses that harm community health and safety know that is inappropriate—that it's not right—so they spend a lot of time trying to convince us otherwise. Early in the fight against smoking, corporate players pushed for individual education and smoking-cessation clinics as viable solutions, understanding that they'd scarcely reduce consumption and profits but could look like they were concerned. They fought policy change at all cost and sold themselves as neighborly good guys. Philip Morris was the poster boy of the good corporate citizen, heavily advertising its support for battered women's shelters.[15] This softened the public perception of tobacco as a destructive industry and garnered consumer confidence—until it was revealed that the company spent more promoting its charitable contributions than it did on the contributions themselves.[16]

Many health-damaging businesses also promote their role as employers and instill fear of layoffs if product demand drops. Coke even touted its affirmative-action agenda, which only arose in response to Martin Luther King Jr. encouraging a boycott of its products (just before his assassination).[17] Maintaining jobs is an important concern, of course, but we don't need jobs that result in cancer, heart disease, and diabetes as significant outcomes. Instead, identifying and helping people transition into jobs that don't produce health-damaging products is the real win-win. In Kentucky, for example, the state government helped move tobacco farmers to new crops and incentivized new markets for them.[18]

Once we accept that there are businesses whose core practices and product lines are fundamentally harmful to health and safety, we can take collective action to protect our communities from further harm. Taking action against harmful business practices can be controversial—but it's needed to prevent needless illness and injury—and health leaders can be catalysts for this kind of action. As Dr. Trevor Hancock says, "Public health is political—always was, always will be. . . . It is not our role to be neutral in these situations. We are not neutral; we are very clearly pro-health, which means we are very clearly opposed to health-damaging activity, no matter the source. If we are not biased, we are not doing our jobs."[19] Part of the solution is to bring communities and consumers together, cultivating a groundswell of activity to control bad businesses and build a movement for change. A variety of strategies can be adopted to protect health, including policy and regulatory action, changing consumer buying practices and norms, strikes, legal action, and grassroots advocacy. And, of course, directing our support—and our purchasing power—toward businesses that promote health not only supports these businesses but also sends a powerful message to health-harming businesses that their practices need to change.

Patti Rundall is policy director of the Baby Milk Action, the UK member of the global network the International Baby Food Action Network (IBFAN). IBFAN has consistently shown over the years how persistent grassroots advocacy and creative, strategic thinking can hold even the largest health-harming business to account. IBFAN, a grassroots network turned worldwide leader for the protection of breast- and formula-fed babies, has led the ongoing international boycott against global baby formula giant Nestlé. Nestlé is continuously called out for its aggressive, and misleading, marketing of baby foods in clear breach of international marketing standards.[20,21] Nestlé's suggestions, for example, that infant formula "protects" babies or its promotion of "breast milk like" formulas are particularly problematic in developing countries where clean water and money are scarce, and breastfeeding is the single most effective preventive measure for ensuring the survival and health of young children.[22] As the World Health Organization states, improved breastfeeding practices could save some 823,000 infant lives annually.[23] For many families and infants, the marketing practices adopted by Nestlé can in fact become a matter of life and death.

IBFAN and other nongovernmental organizations monitor, document, and publicize the violations by Nestlé and all the other formula manufacturers. This "name and shame" approach and the tide of public opinion against Nestlé from the boycott help the public and policymakers understand the importance of regulating corporations. IBFAN has helped more than 100 countries bring in laws that are bringing and end to some harmful practices. But there is still a long way to go. Rundall notes, "Businesses can't be left to regulate themselves. It's not that companies want to deliberately harm health; it's that they have a fiduciary duty to their shareholders to maximize profits. That's the problem. With global sales worth USD 58 billion, baby foods are the fastest growing food sector; it's inevitable that companies will compete for the largest share of the pie and oppose legislation that protects consumers and gets in their way."[24,25] Owning several shares of Nestlé stock herself, Rundall also uses her own voice as a stockholder to drive change from within the company and attends shareholder meetings to point out how shareholders themselves are being misled about the extent of the company's violations and negative reputation. The bottom line for her is that ordinary people and communities can be highly effective in taking on powerful corporations. She says, "This type of action is not dependent on money. Many of the best movements in the world are driven by public outrage, not because someone has written a funding proposal. Indeed, the wrong funding can actually stop people from speaking out as they should."[26]

Rather than trying to settle for a far too elusive "win-win," our collective energies would be better spent on putting the brakes on bad business practices and products and resolving the contradictions in marginal situations, relying on public policy, consumer pressure, and common sense to push for healthy commerce. The other side of progress is praising good businesses and encouraging beneficial practices, products, and business structures that create thriving, sustainable communities, where all elements promote health. Consumers have the opportunity to leverage their purchasing power to incentivize positive businesses and businesses practices. Industry tracks this—why else would Phillip Morris endorse the Vatican exhibit? Enterprising people who understand prevention on the individual level can take effective action on the systems level—breaking through norms and getting people in organizations to think and behave differently. In addition, savvy entrepreneurs and politicians, who understand the value of taking smart risks, can cultivate political will and new ways of thinking and investing in business that advance health rather than illness.

CONTRADICTIONS ON THE ROAD TO INCREMENTAL CHANGE

A colleague I greatly admire called me not long ago to say Walmart was stating, with pride, that it is the largest distributor of organic foods in the United States. Not only that, but it was also heralding its fair labor practices in the organic arena. Shouldn't it be praised for this? It was a dilemma, having just read about Walmart's other newest investment—its state-of-the-art fleet of ocean liners, behemoths that rush across the Pacific from China in just five days, toting much of Walmart's merchandise and certainly not supporting US manufacturing. The vessel clips right back to China—empty—except for the jobs and the money it's taking with it.

Dilemma is the right word. How should we respond when harmful businesses make some improvements to their products or practices? At what point does a business make a bona fide flip to supporting health, and when can consumers trust this? It's a slippery slope when companies try to build credibility by contradicting their standard products and practices. Certainly, on the one hand, Walmart making organics more broadly accessible in a just way benefits its consumers and the organics labor force. On the other hand, touting their organics also gives a false impression of Walmart's overall big-box business model, which is generally anti-health and antilabor,[27] including prohibiting its workers from using their employee discounts toward the purchase of most foods.[28]

While good behavior and healthy products should definitely be encouraged, businesses shouldn't be let off the hook entirely by praising them too quickly—or too much. If a business can go 10 percent of the way toward changing harmful products or practices, we should have our eyes set on the 90 percent that's left. The praise that companies receive for steps in the right direction should be balanced and administered in a way that urges further efforts. And it's only worth doing if the change is highly significant. San Francisco made a bold policy statement, forbidding pharmacies from selling tobacco.[29] I'm impressed by how CVS significantly upped the ante, first by eliminating cigarettes from its nationwide market and then withdrawing from the National Chamber of Commerce to protest the Chamber's endorsing corporate freedom to sell tobacco products worldwide.[30] Clearly this was praiseworthy, although when one walks into their stores, the business model, while no longer including tobacco, still seems to be "come for the medicine; buy the candy and junk food."

So it can be tricky. In 2006 Campbell's Soup received much public praise for lowering the sodium content in its most popular soups by 25 to 45 percent.[31] However, in 2011 Campbell's Soup announced it was increasing sodium levels about halfway back up again in thirty-one of their Select Harvest line soups in an effort to boost sales and improve taste.[32] Coke, on the other hand, while pledging to no longer advertise its products directly on TV programs aimed at children, has instead shifted its efforts to reach children online (to great success).[33] As each of these examples highlights, it is important to be sure that otherwise praiseworthy efforts don't obscure underlying contradictions in a corporation's alignment with health. Hard as it is, we have to project a nuanced message. We don't want to diminish incentives for businesses to be more health supportive by being critical no matter what they do. But companies should be making visible and significant strides to resolve the contradictions, and we must hold much of our applause until they near the finish line or at least until we are confident they are really trying to get there.

ANCHORING NEIGHBORHOODS

I recently visited Detroit's historic Eastern Market neighborhood, an area that had declined with economic travails and disinvestment. A non-profit supported by entrepreneurs and civic leaders has been revamping this market, using it as an anchor in revitalizing the entire neighborhood. In a way, this is one of many examples of what's emerging as the seeds following a fire. When fire destroys a forest, it's a great tragedy; yet certain seeds can flourish in the aftermath once the fire clears. The Eastern Market's original commerce centered on slaughterhouses and hay, but it also endures to this day as a significant source of fresh, local produce. The market has renovated its historic buildings and has expanded operations to an adjacent meat market, becoming a bastion of culturally diverse, fresh, healthy foods and local wares.

The energy and creativity spurring this community revitalization have sparked other innovations. One local business, creatively named Drought, has used a new method of packaging cold-pressed juice so it stays fresh for one month, not a day and a half.[34] *Interest in this product has spread beyond Detroit, with interest from Whole Foods in marketing it across the country. It's part of a whole movement of small entrepreneurs, local businesses, micro loans, and big dreams. The feeling of uplift, purpose, and well-being is infectious—in a good way, because it's based on youthful vitality, entrepreneurism, innovation, and delicious surprise.*

Fortunately, numerous business efforts are easy to support and are clearly moving in the direction of health. In many cases, supporting local community-based businesses emerges as one of the best ways to take back our health, environment, and economy. It's more appealing to shop in small local stores, uncover unique handmade crafts, and talk with the farmers at the farmers' markets. Often, a community-focused business takes good care of its workers, offers high-quality goods and services, and is socially responsible. I especially like small, family-run enterprises. Many are innovative and create middle-class jobs. Local businesses also provide character, personalized service, and stability for communities— enhancing both the physical environment of the neighborhood and social interactions. Government support for local efforts can include tax breaks, subsidies, and policy supports, so small businesses can better compete with big business while maintaining their high standards and values.

Nearly all communities are also home to larger institutions that can play an important role in supporting the overall community environment and keeping smaller businesses afloat. Recently the term "anchor" has emerged to describe the community health–promoting role of institutions that, once established, tend to remain fixed in the same community. Community anchors—including hospitals, universities, and libraries— can exert considerable positive influence on health and local economies through their own practices and policies as employers, purchasers, and neighbors. Tyler Norris, vice president of Total Health Partnerships at Kaiser Permanente, is leading the institution's groundbreaking work in an area it calls "Total Health." As an anchor institution in its hometown, as well as across its footprint, Kaiser has always understood its community responsibility to be commensurate with its role as one of the largest employers, landowners, and service providers. For decades, it has gone beyond the traditional role of a healthcare institution to build health infrastructure in the community by hiring neighborhood youth, supporting local purchasing, powering its facilities with wind and solar energy—creating green jobs in the process—and bolstering sustainable agriculture via grant making and using funders' assets and their purchasing power to strengthen communities. Kaiser not only brought dozens of farmers' markets to its facilities and areas lacking fresh produce, but it also revived a cherished "competitor," the Food Mill, one of the oldest organic markets serving East Oakland. Kaiser has found appropriate ways to reduce and dispose of its toxic waste and has helped reduce community risk by supporting Health Care Without Harm, a pioneer in environmental cleanup of medical waste and, more recently, green purchasing and sustainable food development.

Now Kaiser is redefining health leadership through the Total Health model—increasingly localizing its procurement, sourcing over $1.5 billion per year from women- and minority-owned firms, and helping build a workforce pipeline for youth from vulnerable communities. Now it is looking at ways to extend this sense of community responsibility to every baby born in Oakland. One vision is to partner with other anchor institutions and the City of Oakland in funding a savings account for all local newborns. The Oakland Promise goal is to ensure every child in Oakland graduates high school with the expectations, resources, and skills to complete college and be successful in the career of his or her choice, knowing that quality education is one of the most significant determinants of health and safety. Kaiser understands that this type of health investment will help redress community inequities, build thriving neighborhoods, and yield significant financial returns.

Needless to say, it's appropriate that a healthcare institution is taking this kind of lead, but all anchor businesses, large and small, have a significant role to play in fostering total community health. I was encouraged to learn that San Francisco's Federal Reserve Bank is evaluating ways to position banks as anchor institutions, systematically investing community development funds in local infrastructure that supports health and safety. Even banks can see that aligning health with business, in an equitable, comprehensive way, benefits all community participants. We can extend this notion of Total Health as an anchor for all of our efforts—individual, community, and organizational—to promote holistic, sustainable communities, where health and prosperity flourish.

JSINESS OF HEALTH

y staff members approached me saying, "We have pretty good health insurance for a small nonprofit, but it's really after-the-fact treatment. What about prevention? Why don't we support prevention?" Like every other executive director, I said, "That's a really nice idea, but we can't afford it." After thinking about it, we came up with the notion of a wellness benefit, where every employee has a monthly allowance to spend on a range of wellness activities. I'm glad my staff had the foresight to talk to me about this. Rather than costing money, I now believe it more than pays for itself in improved morale, reduced sick time, and greater engagement in the work.

We all prosper when businesses—small and large—align with health. Benefitting from a healthy workforce, companies can focus on leveraging the many opportunities that spring from preventing illness and injury and investing in community betterment—boosting short-term gains and securing long-term viability. Healthy communities in turn attract additional business investments, creating a virtuous cycle. With increased demand, businesses can reinvest more in innovative research and development, strengthening competitiveness, bolstering employment, and increasing discretionary spending. From a community perspective, there's more money for infrastructure—improving parks, roads, and schools—and for goods, like classroom computers and nutritious school lunches. A study released in 2016 even confirmed that stock portfolios that invested in business that were recipients of the C. Everett Koop National Health Award—bestowed upon businesses with effective workplace health promotion programs—"significantly outperformed the Standard & Poor's (S&P) 500 Index over the past 14 years."[35]

Businesses work very hard to build positive impressions and relationships with consumers because these impressions directly impact their bottom lines. And just as consumer demand has contributed to a growth in more ethical, healthy business practices and products, consumers can demand greater commitment to authentic health and safety on the part of all businesses. For example, the advent of Benefit Corporations (B Corps) means that mission-driven companies serving the triple bottom-line—people, profits, and the planet—no longer need to be at odds with corporate bylaws. Shareholders agree to revise bylaws, allowing decisions to consider the employees, the community, and the environment as well as shareholders. B Corps should meet stringent ongoing requirements in all of these areas. Truly defining good corporate citizenship, they establish a different set of values for consumers and investors.

When individual and corporate interests synchronize with community well-being, the resulting goods and services are more aligned with the health of communities. Norms are steadily shifting such that policies, rules, and ethics guiding acceptable business practices are creating expectations that business needs to be a core community contributor. Working together, what's good for business is good for health.

[10]

HEALTHCARE: A WIDE-ANGLE LENS AS WELL AS A MICROSCOPE

THE BEST MEDICAL CARE IN THE WORLD

I was sitting in an outdoor café in San Francisco with a friend. A doctor my friend knew happened to come by, and she stopped to join us. We chatted for a while, and as I talked about my work, the doctor burst into tears. She'd had a hard day, she confided, diagnosing a patient with severe diabetes. In breaking the news to him, she explained that besides taking his medication, he'd need to start taking better care of his health. The man listened and nodded as she talked about going for regular walks and consuming more fruits and vegetables. Sadly, they both knew he couldn't follow her advice; he worked long hours and returned at night to an unsafe neighborhood where the only nearby food sources were convenience and liquor stores. The same community conditions that triggered his disease would also thwart his efforts to manage it. "When he walked out the door," she confessed, "I felt like a hypocrite, like I had failed him. I felt powerless."

More than anyone, healthcare practitioners are aware of the inevitable outcomes when prevention is largely ignored. They experience the impact of healthcare systems overburdened by people suffering from illnesses and injuries that they were set up to suffer. It's no accident the young doctor felt she had "failed" her patient; the nation's doctors and allied health professionals have become stymied in their efforts to compensate late in the game for factors largely beyond their purview. The current system is rigged against them, and all of us.

But the doctor doesn't need to feel powerless. As we increasingly understand the critical ways our community environments shape health, new strategies have emerged around the roles healthcare can play in supporting improvements to these environments. The most significant opportunity is a shift toward *community-centered health*—combining access to high-quality healthcare with prevention strategies that reduce the frequency and severity of injury and illness in the first place. (Dr. Jack Geiger, discussed in a previous chapter, was an early innovator of this movement.) Community-centered health leverages the best of healthcare—its practice, ethics, and innovations—and the deep commitment and passion that healthcare providers bring to building and restoring health. This focus is particularly important for advancing well-being among those who currently experience the worst health and safety outcomes as a result of living in communities that have been systematically disenfranchised and neglected.

But the promise of a community-centered health system isn't just for low-income families—a broader approach to health can benefit everyone. Even affluent families also have to contend with a constellation of health-diminishing factors: unhealthy products, environmental disasters, and fast-paced streets. So a system that emphasizes not just capital "H," capital "C" Health Care but also embraces a broader definition of health where parks, schools, and housing, for instance, are all recognized as important parts of keeping everyone healthier and better off would benefit affluent and low-income families alike.

Generally, US healthcare providers don't engage with underlying community health influencers in the course of treatment, even though modifying these upstream factors can exponentially decrease the number of people who get sick and are injured and further can improve end of life and decrease the severity and complexity of common conditions. Additionally, clinicians have not typically been taught or encouraged to see this as their job, since community conditions fall outside their scope of practice. Rather, their perspective—formed by graduate medical education, the culture of modern medicine, and healthcare delivery and payment systems—centers primarily on treating individuals who are already sick or injured. Since healthcare professionals are widely venerated as the experts on everything related to health, this focus on "sick care" deeply influences our societal views on how to foster health.[1,2]

A significant number of people in the United States believe, even if their own personal experiences might not always support it, that ours is the best healthcare system in the world.[3] In some ways this is quite true—though primarily for some diseases and some people. For the most part, the US healthcare system excels in specialty care for acute conditions—training world-class specialists to administer the finest treatments for complex, expensive procedures, such as liver transplants and open-heart surgeries. Considering my own family's history and experiences with illness, especially the heroic support of doctors with my mother's cancer—including skillful integration of key pharmaceuticals and the benefits reaped from ever-emerging innovation and technology—how could I not be grateful and deeply appreciate the unparalleled ingenuity and expertise of the US medical system?

At the same time, hiding in plain sight is the stark reality that some health outcomes in the United States lag behind many industrialized, and even some developing, nations.[4,5] For this reason, some international studies rank our overall medical care thirty-eighth in the world.[6] US primary and acute-care systems need improvement in many critical areas: long wait times for emergency and other services, rushed medical visits, high rates of medical errors and complications, insufficient coordination among an increasing number of specialists, low rates of job satisfaction among doctors and nurses, a shortage of general practitioners, facilities and practices reflecting illness not wellness, and persistent inequities in access and quality of care. Still, and quite interestingly, polls consistently confirm that most US residents value and trust their medical care.[7]

While this public faith in our current system is understandable when applying a certain treatment lens, it's also rooted in the popular misconception that health derives primarily from treatment. Overreliance on after-the-fact care as the solution also distracts us from responding to a critically pressing question: How do we reduce the need for clinical care, by keeping people healthier and safer? Many critical health conditions—including diabetes, asthma, cardiovascular, injuries, and HIV—develop more or less frequently based on the circumstances of the environments in which people live.[8,9] Similarly, when we get sick, the likelihood of recuperating depends not only on medical treatment but also on how and where we live. Our approach to health is out of sync with today's chronic, often preventable, health concerns, which call for a wide-angle lens as well as a microscope.

Appropriately, our health system takes heroic measures to save people's lives (and in fact much of our healthcare spending and efforts occurs for end-of-life measures), yet—inappropriately—it fails to emphasize a whole host of practical steps that would prevent injuries and illnesses. As a nation, we willingly try extreme experimental procedures, yet we spurn promising, very low-risk efforts to advance prevention, saying we aren't sure they will always work.[10] With heroic efforts, cost is frequently not a barrier; yet, with prevention, too often decision-makers in healthcare ask, "Is it cost saving? What is the return on investment?"

Thankfully, this medical treatment–centric view of health is changing. Spurred by the nation's attention to healthcare reform, there is growing momentum for ~~strategies based on *health* needs rather than on *healthcare* needs alone~~. Increasingly, in US healthcare circles, one hears conversations about addressing physical, social, and economic conditions in areas such as housing, safety, and food—community elements that can either increase or diminish people's need for medical care and influence health outcomes for better or worse. While treatment and prevention are often considered separate, creating a twenty-first-century health system requires a comprehensive approach whereby treatment and prevention are complementary and mutually sustaining. As prevention efforts improve neighborhood conditions and support structures, the need for costly urgent care decreases, and disease management strategies become more effective and affordable. Healthcare providers have more time to tend to those in most critical need while also promoting health. At the same time, as healthcare institutions focus more on health, they reinforce the importance of wellness and of improving both community and medical environments. Creating a twenty-first-century health system is within our reach.

THE WALLET BIOPSY AND THE BUSINESS OF MEDICAL CARE

In our current system, the first hurdle everyone has to clear is the *wallet biopsy*: the insurance coverage cards we're able to produce from our wallets, or not, when we walk into a healthcare facility determine which services we qualify for, the extent of our coverage, and the quality and cost of those services. Despite tremendous coverage expansions through the Affordable Care Act, millions of people in the United States—primarily low-income, working-class, and populations of color—still fail this wallet test, or only pass minimally.[11]

We risk a lot but gain nothing when we both fail to provide accessible healthcare coverage to all and neglect to invest in prevention strategies that improve community conditions. Consider the consequences of uninsured restaurant workers (who are unlikely to have paid sick days) handling food while suffering from untreated communicable diseases. Sooner or later, our healthcare system is forced to reckon with people's unmet health and safety needs, often by providing very costly emergency care that comes too late to be of significant benefit. And, far too frequently, the nation's jails and prisons serve as the healthcare facility of last resort, providing "care" funded by the public's taxes and insurance pools.

So the insurance test is both a problem unto itself and an indicator of a system in which profit and the bottom line frequently serve as a barrier to health. Sometimes this business orientation aligns well with quality service and treatment, but often it doesn't. The business of healthcare drives the system, with its focus on maximizing financial returns—especially short-term gains. This profit paradigm is the reason why health insurers have traditionally resisted providing coverage to those with previous conditions and why they define healthcare as narrowly as possible, often excluding or significantly limiting access to vital services such as vision, dental,[12] and mental health. This same profit paradigm has led to healthcare institutions permitting the investment of nearly $2 billion of their immense financial reserves in fast-food company stocks,[13] despite being aware that fast food undermines health. Prioritizing profit over health explains why lobbyists representing medical, insurance, and pharmaceutical interests shell out $1.4 million *every day* to maintain the status quo, thereby protecting their lucrative business interests.[14]

As long as major healthcare industries are making landmark profits, as they are now, there will not be sufficient incentive for large-scale change. Regulations protect and insulate the financial beneficiaries of our healthcare system, and the confluence with medicine's prestige and credibility can make positive change difficult. As a result, the impetus for shifting away from the current business model of healthcare has to come from all of us as consumers.

It's unquestionably in our interest, financially and health-wise. Financially, individuals pay dearly for increasingly limited medical services, and businesses bear a huge burden of costs associated with health insurance, lost productivity, and workers' compensation. Our nation allocates $1 of every $6 of our gross domestic product (GDP) for healthcare,[15] spending almost all of this—96 percent—on after-the-fact treatment of illnesses and injuries.[16] Such runaway healthcare costs disrupt our domestic economy, minimize investments in other crucial areas, such as education and social services, and thwart us in the international arena, where other wealthy countries spend a fraction of what we do on healthcare. For example, Australia spends $1 of $11 dollars of its GDP.[17]

Our national approach, at best, tries only to minimize the increase in healthcare costs. In reality, as long as the business of healthcare trumps health itself, goals to improve clinical care and achieve health will remain out of reach and secondary to industry bottom lines. By shifting to a prevention paradigm, our country can spend less, recapture savings, and reinvest those resources in advancing well-being by fostering community conditions that encourage equity, safety, and health.[18,19] It will require different payment mechanisms and different expectations of healthcare's services and roles. As patients—along with advocacy organizations—if we want to see incentives more focused on health rather than profit, we need to speak up to our healthcare leadership, to our practitioners, and to our political representatives.

THE DOCTOR'S DILEMMA

Just as consumers' health and finances aren't served by the current system, neither is the professional well-being of doctors. Most physicians enter the medical profession with a mission to help people. Despite succeeding through the pressure cooker of medical school competition, they're saddled with very costly tuition, yielding high levels of debt and anxiety, which frequently influence their selection of specialty. What's more, billing, record keeping, prescribing, and needing to defend diagnoses to insurance companies—all in speed-up mode—increasingly dominate medical practice. Providers often become discouraged and exhausted, just as they are starting their careers.

Primary care providers, including internists, family medicine practitioners, and pediatricians, have the most responsibility for coordinating care, supporting patients in prevention and wellness, and detecting disease early to minimize impact. As the hub of our healthcare system, these clinicians' jobs are only getting more difficult and stressful. They have to see more patients in shorter time spans, including those recently added to the system, whose prior lack of adequate healthcare and, generally, far more disadvantaged living environments have diminished their health. At the same time, despite the perception that all doctors enjoy inflated salaries, primary care providers, relatively speaking, are comparatively less compensated given the level of coordination and responsibility they bear.[20]

Promoting an expanded, integrated focus on community prevention can, over time, begin to reverse the demands and stress on front-line doctors, who needn't feel that they are powerless. Contributing their wisdom and expertise via community channels, as they treat illness and injury, doctors can lend their credibility and power in speaking up for a new *health system*. Advocating for improved community conditions, they can help increase people's access to healthy environments and to the beneficial lifestyle choices such environments offer. Such a shift in focus better aligns doctors with their primary mission, helps restore their stature, and more effectively mobilizes their understanding of what health really is.

THE HUNGARIAN IMMIGRANT

Several decades ago when I was directing a psychiatric halfway house, I interviewed a woman named Marta who had spent more than twenty-five years at a state hospital for the mentally ill. In the course of our meeting, I discovered that traumatic experiences had landed her there and that she was depressed and distraught in response to her early adolescent experience and history. Having suffered through the Hungarian Uprising of 1956, where tens of thousands were brutally killed and many more badly mistreated, she fled the country as a teen, leaving family, possessions, and her heritage behind.

After escaping to the United States, Marta lost touch with her family and never saw them again. Shocked, isolated, and stressed, she did not have access to any of the community supports that might have enabled her to rebuild her life. And speaking only Hungarian—a language people didn't recognize, so they assumed it was gibberish—Marta was unable to communicate the desperation of her situation. Instead, well-meaning practitioners "rescued" her from the streets and hospitalized her, but they never provided the appropriate supports for her to leave the facility.

When I learned this, I was speechless and outraged. I realized this was a glaring case of mistreatment that was bluntly categorized as mental illness. Marta may have been so initially, but she was then victimized by institutionalization even when she was no longer ill or remotely dangerous to herself or others. Her nearly twenty-five years of confinement was not only unnecessary but a setback, as it weakened Marta's ability to care for herself and thrive. In Marta's case, the lack of understanding that was a byproduct of a well-intentioned but flawed healthcare system resulted in an ongoing clinical diagnosis. In fact, she most needed a framework of support to manage the trauma she experienced in her flight from Hungary.

I helped Marta become a resident of the psychiatric halfway house I directed, which served just over a dozen people who lived there for eight to ten months each. Sweet in nature, Marta had adapted to institutional life without creating a fuss or getting on people's radar, and this learned acquiescence became her lifestyle. As quickly as she learned English, she had also learned the skills of being institutionalized.

Although Marta's trauma was very severe, when placed in a nurturing community environment, she was able to build resilience—an ability to take care of herself and cope with past traumatic events—with the support of a positive peer network. With the help of former residents and the halfway house staff, Marta eventually developed basic self-care abilities and life skills, so she could manage everyday tasks with confidence, ease, and joy. Emotional support from friends was essential, and though she was shy at first, Marta was able to integrate into the halfway house community and become more confident. She was able to move from "what's wrong with me" to "what's happened to me" and *to an increased understanding of what was good about her. Most important, Martha realized she was likeable and that she had the impetus and ability to offer support to others.*

Marta's experience is individually important, but it is also emblematic of the potential improvements needed in the whole health system. Resilience is important for everyone, because we all experience trauma at some point in our lives. At the same time, while trauma, stress, and anxiety are expected parts of life, they are far too common in the United States, due to social and economic inequities—for example, some people face issues such as racial and gender discrimination, chronic unemployment, unstable housing, bullying, and violence. The epidemic of suicides among LGBTQ youth is one such piece of evidence. Stigmatizing LGBTQ youth—whether through messages in popular and social media, bullying by classmates,[21] or statements by friends and family—creates trauma and stress.[22] Many are highly vulnerable youth of color, and the trauma plays out as behavioral health problems and an increased rate of physical and sexual abuse, STDs, incarceration, and murder, as well as suicide.[23]

Healthcare professionals know that issues of trauma, stigma, and anxiety play out in increased physical health symptoms, including overeating or undereating, misuse of substances, and compromised immunity, resulting from discontent rather than well-being. Substance-abuse problems frequently come from self medication for physical and emotional pain. Thus, mental health concerns translate into greater likelihood, severity, and earlier onset of illness and injury. People with mental health disorders and also those with substance-use disorders are among the highest utilizers of clinical services, especially urgent care. A recent study found that people with diabetes used emergency services seven times more often when they also had mental health or substance-abuse issues.[24] As another example, children who face trauma are more likely to develop high blood pressure and elevated cholesterol and are at increased risk for asthma, diabetes, stroke, heart disease, cancer, chronic lung disease, and liver disease later in life.[25] Conversely, physical illnesses have an emotional side, which is why cancer support groups, for example, can be powerfully healing. To ignore or deprioritize the needs of those facing mental health issues is both uncaring and unwise, reflecting a short-sighted, fragmented viewpoint and furthering the sense of hopelessness, stigma, and shame that people too often experience.

Providers can benefit patients by simultaneously addressing mental health conditions as part of standard clinical practice and by identifying community-wide solutions. It became very clear to me, in directing a halfway house, that people need opportunities both to garner skills related to self-care, work, and social interactions as well as to share their unique issues and needs in a welcoming environment. Of course, the complement to encouraging personal and social supports is cultivating thriving living conditions, where people have access to jobs, transportation, housing, resources, services, and safety. As our healthcare paradigm continues to shift toward fostering health, clinical leadership and practitioners should respond to the community conditions that can either diminish or enhance physical *and mental* well-being. In many cases, the same approaches that improve physical health are also responsive to and advance mental health at a community level.

When I served as the chair of the California-wide mental health directors' prevention committee in the 1980s, I helped devise a campaign called Friends Can Be Good Medicine to highlight the simplicity and importance of social inclusion, peer support, and solidarity among neighbors, friends, and family, especially during difficult times. Positive results reported by counties that put this campaign into place included greater empathy and ability to appreciate commonalities, as seen in part by an increase in peer support groups, twelve-step programs, and cancer survivor groups across the state.

Friends are, indeed, good medicine, but more globally one might say the notion of "medicine" gives the wrong impression, since it's not primarily about treating sickness but reducing and preventing it. At Prevention Institute we now have an initiative we call Making Connections—connections might be described as the "probiotics" that bolster resilience and personal capacity and reduce trauma, stress, and mental fatigue. Expanding this approach to the community, fostering empathy rather than stigma multiplies the effect. Cultivating a society where people care for themselves and each other, embracing differences and focusing on what they like about themselves and one another is key. Working together, communities and healthcare providers need to encourage all aspects of mental health prevention. When the positive personal, interpersonal, and community dimensions are mutually interwoven, people can flourish, engage meaningfully, and succeed with dignity.

Fifteen years later, when I ran into Marta on the street, she was still doing well. Over time, with support and an increased sense of self-confidence, she developed a deeper understanding of herself and the emotional complexities she had faced. Eventually, she gained a level of mastery that allowed her to work with other patients as a nurse's aide. Living independently, she became personally well-adjusted, capable, and proud of her ability to provide nurturing for others.

OUR TREATMENTS ARE KILLING US

I was sitting in my cabin in the country late one evening, writing. I had chest pain, which I attributed to something I ate and proceeded to ignore. When I noticed my left arm and shoulder were aching with radiating pain, I wasn't really alarmed; I am left-handed, and maybe I'd done something to strain a muscle. I even ascribed it to the poor ergonomics of my desk setup. When the pain didn't abate, I started to wonder if I was in my usual pattern of denial and if, in fact, I should be concerned about my symptoms. I finally decided I'd better go to the nearest hospital, which was about an hour away.

When I announced my complaint to the staff in the emergency department, they treated it as an emergency. They got me onto a bed and put nitroglycerin on my tongue, before even drawing blood to see if there was a concern. Once the initial blood work came back, they told me it looked like I was fine—no heart attack. Then I started to feel nauseous and dizzy, and when I reported it, the doctor looked at my monitor and started shouting for assistance. Needless to say, I was scared; I feared I was going from not having a heart attack to having one.

The doctor yelled, "Hurry, he's going Brady"—short for bradycardia—and I was given an IV. Maybe it was the fluids, or maybe it was my anxiety protecting me, but my heart rate and blood pressure both rebounded. I eventually learned, as did the emergency department staff, that you don't give nitroglycerin to a patient without carefully monitoring blood pressure. It turned out I was one of a small minority that is allergic to it, and the precipitous drop in my blood pressure that it caused could easily have led to brain damage, stroke, or death.

The word *iatrogenic* is an odd one until one knows what it means—and then it's scary. The new field of iatrogenic medicine deals with the problems arising from healthcare itself. Iatrogenic causes of injury, illness, or death include procedural and medical errors, hospital-acquired infections and diseases, as well as complications from medications—ranging from anticipated side effects to interactions from multiple drugs and improper usage. This is by no means a rare occurrence.

The shocking prevalence of medical errors came to the public's attention with the 1999 publishing of *To Err Is Human,* a groundbreaking report from the Institute of Medicine that exposed the full extent of this major health challenge.[26] In 2013, another article was published in the *Journal of Patient Safety,* one that found that at least 210,000—and probably more than 400,000—people are killed each year by medical error, and that ten or twenty times that number are "seriously harmed."[27] If deaths due to medical error were classified and tracked as a specific cause of mortality, they would qualify as the third most common cause of death in the United States, killing more people than conditions such as unintentional injuries, Alzheimer's disease, and diabetes.[28]

Some of these healthcare-related illnesses and deaths are caused by the approximately 722,000 "hospital acquired infections," each year, more than half of which occur outside the intensive care unit.[29] Furthermore, adverse drug experiences (ADEs) are the most common iatrogenic illness. Approximately 750,000 people are injured or die each year in hospitals from ADEs, at a cost of up to $136.8 billion.[30] ADEs are more likely to occur in the elderly, Black, and rural populations.[31] And these numbers, though large, do not capture the negative impact of prescription drug misuse and overdose.

For all these potential pitfalls, medication and medical care are blessings. When we suffer and the treatment cures us, there's a sense of unmitigated relief. At the same time, our medical system needs to respect the potential for harm that prescription and over-the-counter drugs carry, ensuring they are adequately tested before approval and administered carefully once approval is secured. (And, of course, made affordable so they reach those who need it.) Iatrogenic problems are another reason preventing illness and injury should be a primary focus of attention and resources.

DRUG ADS—THE SIDE EFFECTS COME WITH UPBEAT MUSIC

I was excited to visit Tanzania for the first time. Before I departed, I had to see a tropical medicine specialist to get a required inoculation for yellow fever. While I was at his office, the doctor reminded me about malaria pills. Since I already had contracted malaria during my last trip, the doctor told me it was even more important to protect myself against further mosquito bites. A new, improved drug had been developed, and only a handful of people had side effects, he said.

The following weekend, a day before leaving, I had dinner with friends. A guest I hadn't met before heard I was going to Africa and said in no uncertain terms that I should avoid the malaria drug at all costs: "Whatever you do, don't take it." She was adamant about its terrible mental health side effects, which she said had come on years ago when she visited Africa and persisted still. Years later, she said, her nerves were still affected and her anxiety persisted. Her ada-mancy and strained verbal tone made me question her judgment; she seemed to be on a personal mission to get me to not take it, yet she didn't even know me. I ignored her advice and took the medication anyway.

A week later, I awoke in the middle of the night in a hotel in a game reserve. The power was switched off every night after midnight, so everything was pitch black. It was absolutely still. I was very frightened but had enough of my wits about me to try and understand why. Not a bad dream, not a memory, not a worry. The fear came and went in waves, from bad, but bearable, to very bad. My entire body was shaking and yet, in a unique sensation, I was aware the anxiety wasn't in my head—only coursing through my body. I understood sud-denly and clearly that it was pure physical fear, not fear of something in par-ticular. I tried to read with a flashlight to distract myself, but I was too anxious to concentrate.

The waves of fear came and went. I felt better in the daylight, but by then I was very exhausted and unsettled. At some point, I realized it had to be the malaria drug. Although I eventually stopped taking it, the fear stayed with me for days and returned intermittently—though not as intensely—for several years. Having previously suffered through malaria, I realized my reaction to the drug was comparatively worse. The entire trip had been completely marred. Other longer-term travelers I met laughed at the notion that the medication "rarely" had side effects. In nearly every group of more than three or four, it seemed at least one person had a similarly bad reaction.

The drug company that manufactured the drug claimed that its use caused serious psychiatric side effects in only 1 in 10,000 people. In keeping with the industry standard, the company defined "serious" as hospitalization, long-term disability, or death. With potentially a billion dollars of investment at stake in any given drug, pharmaceutical companies often focus on the effects they want to see and worry less about side effects.

In fact, in 2000, just three years into the approval of direct-to-consumer marketing of medications on TV, the Government Accountability Office estimated that after viewing a pharmaceutical ad on TV, 8.5 million people in the United States asked their physicians for a specific prescription drug associated with that ad.[32] And research shows that doctors are more likely to prescribe particular brands to patients who ask for them.[33]

Adverse reactions to medications are increasingly common, especially when providers combine drugs, use them in an off-label way, or aren't fully aware of the other medications their patients are taking. Clerical errors, resulting in the wrong drugs or mistakes in dosage, are an additional factor. The result can at times be an uncharted chemistry experiment in patients' bodies. Risks and side effects are built in. Additionally, prescription drug misuse by individuals is involved in 1.4 million visits to emergency departments each year,[34] with over 20,000 deaths in the United States related to prescription drug use every year.[35] Prescription drug addiction is also contributing to the devastating opiate drug epidemic in the United States.

My nitroglycerin incident was a mix of pharmaceutical side effects and medical error. I was lucky and didn't lose what I have come to call the "medical lottery." I use this term because every serious medical interaction comes with significant risks. Medical interventions and drugs are a lottery that we benefit from having the opportunity to play, when needed. However, we also have a realistic threat of losing, so we're better off not playing unless it's absolutely necessary. We all face illness at some time, but prevention is our trump card.

REDUCING THE FREQUENCY
OF PLAYING THE MEDICAL LOTTERY

Common sense tells us that focusing on one person at a time after people are already sick or injured is neither the best nor most efficient way to improve health. In fact, healthcare practitioners and institutions are the first to acknowledge that it's time for a different way of working, one that is no longer characterized by harried providers, overcrowded facilities, avoidable medical errors, or reimbursement policies that incentivize sick care over prevention. Moving beyond the limits of the current healthcare system necessitates a paradigm shift toward a more comprehensive approach to health that more fully meets the needs of practitioners and consumers alike. This requires integrated interventions at the federal, state, and regional levels as well as in the day-to-day practices of healthcare institutions.

Encouragingly, the health system is starting to shift in the right direction. While change at this massive scale happens slowly—at times even imperceptibly—the importance of addressing community conditions and the national structures that shape health is increasingly reflected in the healthcare ethos. The unit of measurement is steadily moving from one of individual patient health to one of population-wide health. Emerging innovations in healthcare payment and service delivery are creating a framework for achieving higher quality care at lower cost.

While the incremental progression in our health system's mindset is undeniable, it won't be as far reaching as we all want—and deserve—unless we deliberately coalesce the changes underway into a new vision for a community-centered approach to health. As is often the case with large-scale social norms change, the local level holds great promise for fostering the innovations needed. There is a long track record of advocacy and leadership among healthcare providers, resulting in substantial, life-saving community changes. For example, using back-door diplomacy to leverage his clout in the community, Dr. Bob Sanders garnered local and then state and federal support for mandatory car-seat laws to prevent children from dying in car crashes.[36] Dr. Mervyn Silverman led the San Francisco Health

Department in closing local bathhouses in the early days of the AIDS epidemic to prevent the spread of HIV.[37] And Dr. Deborah Prothrow-Stith's experiences working with youth at Boston City Hospital and in community settings gave her the insight and courage to say, "Violence is a preventable health issue that we can change"[38] and to organize the community to start achieving such change.

Each of these healthcare leaders intuitively understood that a community-wide focus is necessary, and more local healthcare institutions are stepping outside the clinic walls to support community-wide changes.

Just down the street from me, a neighbor in Oakland's Chinatown was run over and killed at a crosswalk. Staff at Asian Health Services (AHS) realized that pedestrian safety, especially for older people and people with disabilities, was a major health issue in the community. Taking a hard look at the surrounding neighborhood conditions, AHS found that the combination of traffic density, local demographics, street design, and high pedestrian volume greatly elevated the risk for injury and death. Solutions existed; they just needed to be put into place. Youth advocacy and leadership groups within AHS gathered data, mapping and documenting pedestrian vehicle injuries by location. Reaching outside clinic walls, AHS assembled a diverse coalition, including traffic and urban planners, architects, law enforcement, business and local officials, and various neighborhood groups. They held public meetings and spoke at community events, encouraging residents to become involved in the decision-making process. Coalition activity led to redesigning the intersection and traffic flow patterns to improve safety and reduce the probability of injuries and fatalities. The community called the new system the "Oakland Scramble," where vehicles all stop while people cross and people all wait while vehicles take their turns. As a result of these changes, dangerous pedestrian–vehicle encounters at that intersection dropped by as much as 50 percent.[39]

AHS went on to join an even broader set of community partners, launching a successful economic and environmental justice campaign to renew Oakland's Chinatown. Receiving an environmental justice grant from the transportation department and leveraging coalition members' relationships with merchants and politicians, they revitalized the economically depressed commercial district, made further safety improvements, and addressed the unfair plan to route high-polluting diesel trucks through Chinatown, which would have undermined renewal efforts and jeopardized the community's health.

Far exceeding traditional expectations of a healthcare organization, AHS embodies principles and practices that could become core to a new norm for healthcare. By expanding its analysis and focus beyond its own individual patients, AHS demonstrates how healthcare can be responsive to neighborhood needs and contribute to population-wide transformative change. The Prevention Institute coined the term "community-centered health homes" to capture the possibilities when healthcare takes on a community emphasis and to encourage the widespread adoption of this approach. A community-centered health home looks for cues about what underlies its patient's illnesses and injuries and identifies the specific conditions and places where these conditions are generated. At its core, it is a healthcare organization that not only acknowledges that community factors affect patient health outcomes but also actively participates in improving them.

St. John's Well Child and Family Center in South Los Angeles has been on the forefront of community-centered health for more than two decades. When clinicians at St. John's noted scores of patients with skin diseases, insect and rodent bites, cockroaches in their ears, and lead poisoning, they realized that substandard housing conditions were likely the underlying factor and that just treating the resulting problems without getting to the underlying conditions would only lead to repeat visits, not only for these patients but also for others facing the same conditions. Creating a specific intake form to ask patients about their housing conditions, the clinic staff confirmed their hunch and pinpointed the problem. St. John's providers then formed a partnership with community-based organizations working on affordable housing and legal rights—advocacy to tackle the problem at its roots. By sharing clinical data and its implications with its coalition partners, St. John's not only helped individual patients improve their living conditions but also helped catalyze a community-wide campaign to address inadequate housing. As a result of the coalition's joint efforts, landlord compliance, residents' living conditions, and patient health outcomes all improved.[40]

Like AHS, the staff, clinicians, and leadership at St. John's understand that treating individual symptoms, patient by patient, is no longer sufficient. Instead, they are working to reverse widespread health-eroding conditions, as well as their physical and emotional aftermath. They also understand, and feel the need to address, how these conditions stem, to a large extent, from racism and poverty. President and CEO Jim Mangia says, "We feel very strongly that health is a fundamental human right. If you're talking about health, you're talking about more than healthcare. Our approach is comprehensive and holistic."[41]

Cincinnati Children's Hospital has undertaken something similar by using geographic clinical data to determine where community-wide changes can be imposed to reduce clinical needs. The Cincinnati researchers identified asthma "hot spots" in their city, which showed up particularly in low-income neighborhoods. Health leaders realized they could do more to help children by focusing on what was leading to the occurrence of asthma in the first place. Soliciting help from the health department and the legal aid society, the hospital went after the landlords and property managers to rectify what it called "an outbreak of poor quality housing." Robert Kahn, director of the hospital's Community Health Initiative, says, "You can pick up patterns about social problems and contribute to the community solving them. It's a way to bear witness to the impact on a child's health and then look for the cure upstream . . . the power has to rest with formal and informal leadership in the community."[42]

Thus, a community-centered health homes approach allows healthcare providers to apply the standard medical protocol—assessing symptoms, making a diagnosis, and recommending a treatment plan—to a community setting. The providers ask: Why do many people in a certain area have the same illness or injury? What are their air, soil, and water conditions like? Is there a history of street violence? Do they have access to affordable fresh food? Can they walk and play safely outside? Is housing adequate? Sharing this information directly with a wide range of community partners allows healthcare workers to leverage their considerable knowledge and influence in order to actively engage in improving community conditions.

Jack Geiger, the pioneer of the community health center movement, spoke about the issue this way: "What has happened now, and that is beginning to happen, is that community health centers and indeed hospitals and other health delivery organizations, are going to have to [address social determinants of health] by collaborative efforts with other organizations—with public health agencies, with housing departments, with transportation departments, with county executives—to mount, in collaboration, the same kind of interventions."[43]

BECOMING THE INSTITUTION
THAT WALKS THE TALK

Recently, I visited one of the country's most prestigious healthcare institutions. I was excited to be interviewed for a cutting-edge film on heath and prevention. I rode the elevator up from the parking lot, and when I exited found myself in a small lobby where I was met with vending machines stocked with candy and soda and a fast-food operation selling pastries and junk food. I felt disconcerted by the incongruity.

Alternatively, in Houston, Texas, where nearly half the population is Latino, primary care doctor Ann Barnes worked with community members and hospital executive staff to bring healthy, affordable foods to clinic patients via a farmers' market at the door of the clinic lobby. Barnes worked with Veggie Pals, a small, local nonprofit, to canvass the community to see which fruits and vegetables would be culturally relevant. The program sold more than five tons of food in ten months. The local farmers, not incidentally, also benefitted from the increased demand and growing appreciation for what they provide.

Needless to say, all institutions that have healing as their core mission can and should model wellness in all of their practices and actions. Fostering a healthy environment within a healthcare institution's own walls is one part of the shift toward prevention and healthy community change. Does the institution support health in all its policies? Does it patronize only hotels with healthy conference food, walkable staircases, strong no-smoking policies, and good labor practices? Does it accommodate breastfeeding and provide workplace health in employees?

FROM SICK CARE TO A SYSTEM OF HEALTH

The answers to questions such as "What's a specific model for how our health system should be?" or "What should be in place for our health system to change?" are not simple. Typically, as a new paradigm takes shape, there isn't a single place or element but rather different examples with varying attributes that can be combined to begin to create a new, holistic model. Transitioning from sick care to the promise of a community-centered health system calls for creative leadership, innovative strategies, and renewed training. It takes a team to build a fresh way of working and fully implement all the aspects of this new system. As practitioners train to work in a new way, they begin to better understand their roles. As agencies change their practices, they begin to see the impact and discover what else they can do.

Getting there will take a process of stringing together individual, local successes into broader sustainable efforts. So when we talk about improving our health system, the question we should really ask is, "What can advance the solidification of existing and emerging efforts across the country?" The answer there is easy: vision and leadership at a national level. Local successes, however compelling, require a high-ranking hand to connect them; otherwise they remain nice stories in a book like this one.

So how do we compel leadership to bring about the sweeping change described here? The answer is by creating a groundswell of evidence and efficiency—the sort of undeniable, objective data that appeal to legislators and those with the ability to effect change. When it comes to health, the two quantitative advances that can move the needle are smart measurements and payment systems that encourage implementing the vision.

The term *smart measurements* refers to measuring community conditions and medical conditions to judge how effective our interventions for community conditions are. For example, currently, for asthma patients, clinicians measure individuals' spirometry results and exhaled nitric oxide levels. A health system that emphasized prevention would measure air quality levels in the community as well (or perhaps instead). For patients with diabetes, prevention-oriented measurement would gauge access to fresh produce and safe exercise environments, in addition to in A1C levels.

One potential avenue for implementing smart measurements is e-coding, short for "external cause coding." Developed specifically for injuries and now usually in place in trauma centers, e-codes serve as an adjunct to the coding of the *medical* nature of an injury (the "diagnosis"). A diagnosis by a provider comprises a standardized medical code for a particular disease or injury; e-codes, when they are used, go beyond this medical diagnosis to consider the cause. They specify why a death or injury has occurred (unintentional, self-inflicted, assault), the mechanism of death or injury (fall, automobile crash, etc.), and the place of occurrence of the event (playground, home, specific intersection). Knowing that a woman fractured her left clavicle is useful for a clinical response, but e-code information can provide the prevention clues we need to keep others from suffering similar injuries.

E-codes are used in more hospitals today, ushering in a huge shift in the way healthcare networks collect information. In Nebraska, the state's Health and Human Services Injury Prevention Program has established an injury prevention advisory committee to review e-code data and develop an injury prevention state plan that outlines recommendations for reducing the prevalence and severity of injuries in the state. In California, e-code data have been used to enact legislation to decrease the number of small children that drown (or nearly drown) in pools and spas; to establish mandates for firearm safety in response to youth accidents and suicides; and to create programs that address preventable injuries associated with bikes, motorcycles, senior falls, and child abuse. Similar methodology could be developed for capturing information about chronic illness and preventive measures taken accordingly.

If this level of coding were adopted and applied beyond injuries to all sorts of diseases and medical issues like asthma, heart disease, and diabetes, health professionals would gain significant insights into the community conditions and underlying causes of costly medical conditions. It would open a path to solutions beyond individual treatment in instances where larger patterns emerged and help to shift toward a community prevention approach—especially if adoption of an expanded e-coding system were widespread.

Payment and billing mechanisms are also a critical component to supporting prevention in health. Healthcare providers and institutions must be incentivized to practice prevention, which hasn't happened in the historical "fee for service system." The good news is that we are starting to see momentum for payment mechanisms that emphasize well care instead of sick care. As described earlier, my first prevention position was based on a "capitation" method that paid based on average costs per patient, rather than paying per procedure. In this model, the incentive switched to keeping people from getting sick. As trauma surgeon and former head of the National Highway Traffic Safety Administration Ricardo Martinez once told me, "It used to be I made my money from surgeries, and if I wanted to make more money, I would pray for snow since that meant more broken limbs. But when I get paid the same irrespective of the number of injuries, it makes sense to shovel snow instead."

Fortunately, more approaches that reward wellness have proliferated over the past few years. Health maintenance organizations, because they are paid an overall fee for service, can more easily incentivize prevention efforts. Some current names for similar approaches across the entire health system are "value-based payment" and "global payment." As these approaches take hold and are systematized, and as they impact both insurers and healthcare delivery organizations, prevention will make a lot more sense—and pay better, too.

The Affordable Care Act catalyzed rethinking about our nation's health system for supporters and opponents alike. In addition to its emphasis on care, it created the Prevention and Public Health Fund, resources for communities to collaborate in advancing health. It also created a new government center to advance innovation within the health system. The Center for Medicare and Medicaid Innovation (CMMI) is a central governmental entity for exploring and seeding the kinds of innovation that can help transform the nation's health system overall. CMMI's role is to test ways to help make the medical system to work better, while considering three elements: better care, lower cost, and improved population health. All three legs of the stool are essential: if just one of them is unstable, the entire stool topples.

Fitting a prevention paradigm into a medical approach takes some easing. As it turned out, CMMI was deliberately looking only for changes that showed effectiveness within three years and primarily envisioned such prevention as either clinical services or education (e.g., pap smears and educational brochures). One official, a pediatrician, told me she couldn't imagine prevention efforts saving substantial money—more than they cost to implement—within this brief time period, if at all. So community-oriented prevention approaches, from that perspective, started out mostly off the table. I did see some receptiveness to the idea, however, when I gave proven examples, such as laws requiring passenger restraints and car seats, and no-smoking regulations and taxes, which have saved countless lives and dollars in both the short term and the long run, by preventing unnecessary injuries and illnesses before they occur.

CMMI's growing vision, along with that of healthcare as a whole, is increasingly recognizing and addressing the importance of community environments, primarily from the perspective of what individual patients need and how social services can complement treatment. It has begun to understand and create models for advancing the basic principles of a new way of thinking about health—that efforts must be comprehensive, multifaceted, and beyond brochures. In achieving such innovation, alternative payment systems are a big part of what CMMI is exploring, and as CMMI models become more prevention-oriented, they are helping to change the overall approach of healthcare.

Still, prevention in many cases will benefit an investment before we see outcomes and savings. What Dr. Tony Iton and I call "closing the loop" is an opportunity to seed prevention efforts with relevant taxes and fees that can be applied to prevention. For example, from 1989 to 2008, California invested $2.4 billion—a relatively small portion of the money raised from taxing tobacco and from legal settlements with tobacco companies—and invested it into the California Tobacco Program. This money was spent on efforts to reduce smoking, from supporting community coalitions as they pursued no-smoking policies and practices to hard-hitting media campaigns. According to a 2013 University of California, San Francisco, analysis, the initial $2.4 billion investment saved $134 billion—a 5,500 percent return—thanks to reduced medical expenditures that would otherwise have been needed to treat smoking-related illness.[44]

Unfortunately, very little of this impressive $134 billion in savings has gone back into further efforts to prevent smoking. Given the fruitfulness of the investment, why not invest substantially more? It's time to close this loop and reinvest the savings from prevention into self-sustaining prevention efforts. Wellness trusts are another emerging mechanism that combines funding from diverse sources to create a local, regional, or state pool of funds that can be used to invest in prevention. We've had opportunities to recapture massive prevention savings and create new funding streams for decades and have failed to do so. We need to think big.

ACTUAL CAUSES

In 2010 Dr. Laura Gottlieb, a family and community medicine physician at University of California, San Francisco, poignantly described the dilemma facing healthcare providers when the health system doesn't prioritize community factors: "I have diagnosed 'abdominal pain' when the real problem was hunger; I confused social issues with medical problems in other patients, too. I mislabeled the hopelessness of long-term unemployment as depression and the poverty that causes patients to miss pills or appointments as noncompliance. In one older patient, I mistook the inability to read for dementia. My medical training had not prepared me for this ambush of social circumstance. Real-life obstacles had an enormous impact on my patients' lives, but because I had neither the skills nor the resources for treating them, I ignored the social context of disease altogether."[45]

Now, a few years later, the good news is that creating a twenty-first-century health system that embraces wellness and addresses community conditions through prevention is more within reach. Our talented medical leaders are starting to marshal their credibility and dedication to balance the importance of treating immediate medical concerns with the opportunity to prevent illness and injury in the future. Forward-thinking institutions are demonstrating the possibilities for healthcare to shift its entrenched practices to better align their goals, profit incentives, and external partnerships to further advance health. The progress within the healthcare system—and within communities—arises from changes on the local and federal levels, each supporting one another and furthering the overall momentum.

Ultimately, we have to learn to think differently and more intuitively to create significant, lasting health change. If we could see concepts as interrelated and view health and healing from that perspective, fitting a prevention paradigm into a medical approach wouldn't require so much easing. Dr. Tiearona Low Dog, a Native American medical doctor, shared her moving perspective on this, saying, "My definition of medicine was formed at a young age. I was coming back with my grandmother, from Medicine Lodge, Kansas, where we had attended a pow-wow. She was driving the pickup truck, and at one point she looked over to me and said, 'You know baby, you have to remember that when you were born, you were set on a road, and that road is your medicine road. Everything you do in your life—everything—is medicine, good or bad: the way you think, the way you move in the world, the way you treat other people, the thoughts you think, the food you eat. All of it is your medicine, so think carefully about the way you live your life.' "[46] To this, I would add that the environments in which we live, work, and play are our medicine, and we have a responsibility to those environments as everyone's medicine.

When health and prevention are the primary goals, *everyone* benefits from supportive community conditions, comprehensive preventive care, and full access to quality treatment when it is required. And yet, moving toward a better, fairer, more efficient health system has become quite controversial in US politics. Experts and politicians in the United States have tied themselves in knots over what government's role should be in healthcare, especially at the national level, but it's mostly common sense. It's time to repair partisan relations and ensure that government decisions better represent the people's interest, redirecting policies to protect our mutual well-being and reasserting our fundamental right to health and safety. As we move back toward a national understanding of the need to focus on and invest in health, we must also move from just sick care to prevention. Dr. Tony Iton, a visionary leader in public health and social justice, and physician by training, remarks, "Healthcare is what happens when things go wrong."[47] Prevention is what happens when things go right. It's up to us to spread the word on what is possible—and make sure it's equitable.

[11]

IT TAKES A FLOCK
TO MAKE A BIRD SOAR

ON THE BEACH

It was 2013, and the sign dangling on a thin wire announced the beach ahead was closed due to the federal government shutdown. How do you close a beach? Slinking under the wire, my dog and I headed down the familiar trail, eager to reach one of the few beaches in Northern California where dogs are welcome to run. On a balmy Sunday like this, we'd usually share the expansive crescent cove with many others out playing with their kids and dogs. But hearing that the beaches were closed, most people didn't venture out and accordingly were deprived of a majestic day. At the same time, as the windswept sand swirled free of its usual footprints and I walked alone in an area where many people usually gathered, I felt strangely soothed—nature without people.

Then I witnessed an amazing sight. It looked very much like a seabird that was surfing. Perched on a piece of driftwood that rocked gently on the waves, the seabird spread its wings to maintain balance as it continued shoreward. Then the undertow pulled it backward, and on the next big wave, the beautiful pattern repeated.

Suddenly, I realized, in shock, that this was no dance; it was the awful result of human destruction. The bird was trapped, with its leg wrapped in plastic that had somehow become lodged on the driftwood. Signs everywhere warned of the dangers of the undertow on this beach, but I was tempted to dive in. Realizing the bird was too far out and the water too frigid, I restrained myself.

Another bird swooped down. I thought at first it was curious, but it was attempting to bite the plastic. I watched it try again and again. Then I saw a miracle. The constant pecking by the ensnared bird's flock-mate had finally broken the plastic bond. I heard triumphant caws from the rescue bird and the seabird, which had broken free, as they rose in the air and flew off. The seabird still had a piece of plastic dangling from its leg, but now it could fly. What awaits it, I wondered? Does it have the reserves and resilience to survive?

I felt privileged to witness this: what human negligence can impose on nature (and this bird). Similarly, I was exasperated that political dysfunction had robbed people of the healing tranquility of such a beautiful place. The shutdown interfered with basic sustenance—distribution of vaccines, federal preschool programs, food safety and food stamps, and disability and veterans' medical services[1]—while our huge national security apparatus remained in full swing. What can we do when politicians, who should elevate the well-being of their constituents, so frequently refuse to maintain opportunities for health, safety and well-being because of politics? Like the trapped seabird, we're all caught in a system where preventable tragedies and never-ending rescues are the norm. And all of us, but even more so communities facing discrimination and disinvestment, continue to pay an unbearable, inhumane price.

In 2016 people in Flint, Michigan, were poisoned by lead in the water that their government provided them. Government officials were focused on saving money, and no one was held accountable for the needs or concerns of the local community. The tragedy, and travesty, is that whatever may have been saved initially by diverting the water supply pales in comparison to the cost of trying to restore the health and lives of an entire community—not to mention the emotional and psychological anguish that Flint community members have been unnecessarily forced to endure.

It's critical that the community voices be heard and respected. It is also critical that health be taken into account, and, in this case, a decision to save a pittance had an enormous toll in human as well as financial terms. I wrote about lead in a previous chapter as though it were a historic— though not fully achieved—success, and it's difficult for me to understand how this could still happen in the twenty-first-century United States. Though Flint residents, the majority of whom are Black and nearly half of whom live below the poverty line,[2] complained to officials for a long time about the taste, smell, and look of the water, they were ignored. I don't believe such negligence would have occurred in a wealthier, white community. Every solution relating to health should include a focus on prevention, equity, and the concerns of community members.

MEETING FOR COFFEE

I'm sitting in a sidewalk café writing the conclusion of this book, my dog Faroah at my feet, and thinking about how a focus on prevention is such an important part of ensuring fairness and well-being for everyone. I am reminded of the decades of priceless moments I've savored in such cafes, where I come to clear my head, test-drive new ideas, and enjoy the coffee. I've relished the excitement of too-early morning meetings with the doctors who helped hatch plans for the first countywide smoking bans. Most effective coalitions will be driven by subcommittees, including a steering committee that thinks through direction. I have always found the best steering committees need to be creative and informal, so "a few people for coffee" has been the solution that serves me well. "Let's have coffee" has also been the way I've launched creative partnerships, seeded off-the-record policies, and secured prevention funding opportunities.

I germinated my core ideas and began the Prevention Institute's work in a corner of my house. These were great quarters compared to the broom closet where I had begun the county prevention program. Before long, my entire house became a "prevention factory." With as many as ten people coming daily, we outgrew the house and are now in a building of our own—a physical place in the United States that stands dedicated to quality prevention. The Prevention Institute also strives to bring others together, to be an incubator for innovative thinking and momentum, a space where advocates and professionals from many walks of life collaborate and develop strategies for catalyzing community action and inclusive, equitable policy change. We ask the question: What does it take for health and prevention to become the default—where our attitudes, systems, and structures are hard-wired to foster wellness, to the point where positive health and safety outcomes are the norm?

As I consider where the movement for prevention needs to go, I reflect on the significant progress we've made. It's easy to take past success for granted, especially for those who don't remember what was accomplished. Sweeping legislation was passed controlling tobacco,[3] removing lead and asbestos from products,[4] overhauling highway safety,[5] and mandating use of seat belts and child safety restraints.[6] We have seen a renewed interest in local, sustainable, and fresh food—the food of our individual unique histories but also of the histories of so many diverse friends' neighbors and communities. This is starting to create new employment possibilities and make food policy—from farm to table—more clear and relevant to our daily lives. Considering health as part of planning and design has helped to solve issues of transportation, air quality, and access to healthy food, clean water, and physical activity. Street safety has become a more prominent concern, as cities add bike lanes and consider all forms of mobility. And as concerns about buying local products, cleaner air and water, and encouraging walking and biking in *safe* communities grow, the solutions to these issues are equally responsive to climate change—a good solution solving multiple problems.

Sitting here, I recollect that many outdoor cafés, including the one in which I'm sitting, came about as an unintended consequence of helping to ban smoking in restaurants. In many places, zoning had previously prohibited outdoor cafés. But the smoking bans led to restaurant owners pushing for a compromise—outdoor tables where people could smoke—and, in many communities, elected officials were happy to oblige. That's old history, of course. There is no smoking at any of these tables now, at least not in the cities in the lead on tobacco regulations. Now everyone sees that sidewalk cafés are good for pleasure, business, and community vitality. This is more the case in privileged areas, so creating them in all neighborhoods should become an intentional priority while vigilantly ensuring that these community improvements do not displace current residents. In many cities, such cafés have become the best places to sit with your dog and have breakfast or coffee. How ironic for me to learn that outdoor eating originated in Coney Island, nearly a hundred years before I was born.[7]

When Frederick Law Olmsted designed many of our nation's parks at this very same time,[8] he already knew the community environment was vital to public health and justice. Olmsted was a visionary who understood how the natural and social environments affect all people's well-being. He realized beautiful urban sanctuaries could excite people about city living, so he created park experiences that would be restorative, with a "poetic and tranquilizing influence" amidst the steel and concrete. Olmsted also saw the need for green spaces, where city inhabitants could breathe clean air, conceiving and designing Central Park as "the lungs of NY."[9] To me, Olmsted is one of our unnoticed prevention heroes.

I wonder what it means that we don't, as a nation, recognize prevention heroes. The US cultural perception of heroism often requires addressing an issue after a disaster or at a visible time of crisis. We can shift that perception to understand the heroism of those who work to prevent disaster and suffering; of community members who use limited resources to protect their families and navigate an onslaught of external challenges; of those who challenge discrimination, even when it's not safe or deemed acceptable to do so. Alicia Garza, Patrisse Cullors, and Opal Tometi of the Black Lives Matter movement are heroes because they affirm the value of the lives of Black people as well as those who have had a large role, yet have traditionally been silenced in the movements for civil rights, and demand that people directly engage them and their national action. As Patti Rundall of Baby Milk Action reminds us, "Many of the best movements in the world are driven by public outrage, not because someone has written a funding proposal."[10] Nancy Milio was a hero because she encouraged advancing health by emphasizing the decisions and regulations that could reshape our food supply—clarifying that the Farm Bill was not only relevant but critical. I call this heroism through mobilization, and, as Adrienne Rich states, "I have to cast my lot with those who age after age, perversely, with no extraordinary power, reconstitute the world."[11]

CREATING AN ACCESSIBLE WORLD

I recently took the BART train two stops from my house to see the new Ed Roberts Campus at the University of California, Berkeley. I rode the elevator from inside the transit station straight up to the campus, which by embracing Roberts's vision for design has become one of the world's best examples of universal accessibility. Entering the spacious lobby, I wound up the large spiral ramp, which easily accommodated both wheelchairs and foot traffic. I soon discovered a gurgling fountain that provided individuals with visual challenges with an audible signpost for restrooms and water fountains. Inside the bathroom, I found a sling to help people with physical limitations use the facilities independently.

The campus is a tribute to Roberts's work and a milestone development for groups facing ongoing exclusion, discrimination, and other barriers to accessing resources and opportunities. The campus is a living monument of this global struggle for justice, serving as an urgent reminder of how much further the United States has to go in reversing the institutionalized results of social and health injustices—even as it celebrates Roberts's vision and the access movement's collective achievements within just a few decades' time.

Roberts's triumphs are a beacon for social advocates working in other areas who encounter the same limited thinking. Safety advocates, for example, have been told that preventing violence would be impossible. But, as their achievements have shown, violence is entirely preventable. Many cities nationwide have cut street violence rates in half by building a collaborative prevention approach—investing in and supporting communities, especially those at greatest risk.[12] Sports teams are beginning to focus on confronting norms that encourage traditional power dynamics and expectations of masculinity—pushing back against the notion that violence is a reasonable solution to conflict and that sexual assault is somehow masculine and acceptable.[13,14] Schools are starting to focus on helping students build resilience and overcome trauma.[15] Others will feed off this momentum, modifying such efforts to meet their unique needs and achieve similar success. As reformer John Gardner states, "We are all faced with a series of great opportunities brilliantly disguised as insoluble problems."[16] Many things may still feel "impossible," yet it's time to make a lot of progress.

WHAT YOU CAN DO

Many have asked me what I hope people reading this book will do differently. Clearly, this is not about self-care or selecting the right foods to eat, though these are worthwhile pursuits. *Prevention Diaries* is not about one person at a time. Change often happens when a group of people join together in addressing the community issues that influence health and safety and inspire others to do the same, leading to sweeping changes that can save lives and reduce misery. As I started talking with decision-makers in DC and across the country about how to advance community-wide *health,* it was clear that they weren't hearing ideas like mine very often. The need to address this missed opportunity was one of the reasons for writing *Diaries*—we all need to understand and emphasize the notion of "in the first place," and we all need to speak up for the importance of changing the underlying determinants to those that advance health rather than illness, that advance fairness rather than inequity.

You, as the reader, have unique opportunities to get involved in supporting your family and community's health and safety. It's a matter of noticing health triggers and taking whatever actions are feasible to encourage health and safety to flourish. This can be as simple as paying attention to children playing on your street or connecting with neighbors to organize a block party. Ask whether your child's school provides nutritious lunches, free water, and healthy vending machine options. Is the schoolyard equipment safe? What does your school do to stop bullying and keep children emotionally safe? Can you and other parents provide effective input to administrators and the local school board as a next step when needed? What changes might be possible in your workplace that could support employee and community health? You can ratchet up the activity from there, according to your capacity. Team up to make sure your local parks are fully functional, accessible, and safe. Engage in efforts to bring nutritious, culturally desirable foods to your neighborhood, and, if you can broaden your engagement further, consider how to use your connections and resources strategically, build networks within your areas of influence, and help shape policies and practices within your professional organizations and places of worship. As Amelia Earhart said, "The most difficult thing is the decision to act; the rest is merely tenacity." [17] As the general public joins in promoting advocacy, wellness efforts will snowball, norms will shift, and communities will flourish.

INSISTING ON HEALTH

Further tilting the healthcare paradigm toward health is part of the norms shift. The potential for a major transformation of healthcare to meaningfully include prevention is looking ever more promising, but it depends on the public and decision-makers constantly insisting we need prevention, innovation and sustainability. Awareness of the social determinants of health has taken hold, so now it's a question of trying to provide practical and significant ways that medical practice can expand beyond its conventional efforts, understanding that, for many patients, a prescription for housing or healthy food is the most powerful one that a physician could write and that it only becomes fully effective when we look at housing or healthy food overall, not just for that one patient.

The key point is that we can't succeed if we only make changes one person at a time.

A colleague tells the story of two friends walking along a beach covered in stranded starfish. One friend notices them but keeps walking, while the other stops and hurls a starfish as far out into the ocean as he can. "Why bother?" asks the friend who had continued walking. "Didn't you see how many starfish have washed ashore? Just saving one won't make any difference." "Well, it will to the starfish I saved," replies the other friend.

"It's a great story with an important moral," states my colleague. Then he made a strong remark, "The problem is it's been used to justify weak strategy." He went on to say, "When people say, 'If we can just save one life, it's worth it,' it sounds to me like a failed program." I agree with him, in a way. Saving each life is crucial, but when engaged in healthcare work, it is insufficient to remain satisfied with simply saving that single life, because the beach is still covered in dying starfish. It is important to probe more deeply, asking, "What are the factors contributing to this issue? Why is this happening in the first place? What can be done to prevent others from needing to be saved?"

Healthcare's tendency to focus on one patient at a time after the fact should be expanded, so efforts are also directed toward improving the community determinants of health in the first place. I underscore George Albee's saying, "No epidemic can ever be resolved by paying attention to the affected individual." Change will come from local communities and then bubble up to statewide and national solutions. As these innovations expand into a national vision, healthcare transformation will be well on its way. With health and prevention as the primary goals sparking this transformation, *everyone* will benefit from supportive community conditions, comprehensive preventive care, and full access to quality treatment when it is required.

REAL IMPACT

People often ask how we can measure the impact of prevention if we can't see it. I respond that we *can* measure prevention over time in terms of lives saved and money saved. No-smoking policies and tobacco taxes have resulted in half as many smokers in California, for example. (And in every other state we see similar though usually less dramatic declines.) The year after California passed a motorcycle helmet law there was a huge drop in head injuries. While these are just two examples, they represent a great many people who won't face disease or injury, who won't suffer or die, and who probably don't fully recognize how prevention policy and practice have saved their lives.

Failure to act and missed prevention opportunities come at great cost. Without full commitment to health and prevention from our elected officials and in the face of the pervasive sale of products that harm our well-being, many areas of greatest achievement have slipped or reemerged as areas of inequity. For example, while initial successes dramatically slashed rates of smoking, lung cancer, and tobacco-related fires, tobacco is still the number-one killer in the United States, especially in communities that are deliberate targets of heavy marketing, which are invariably the ones experiencing chronic stress—communities of color and Native American communities, people living at or below the poverty line, and LGBTQ communities.[18,19] This isn't by accident. Big Tobacco's marketing deliberately targets the communities and populations they know have the least amount of support and resources. Our nation's most vulnerable pay with their lives, yet they have more limited access to healthcare, including smoking cessation services and tobacco prevention programs.[20]

As we advance prevention, we need to urgently address inequities. Efforts should not only focus on immediate issues but also, more important, on underlying dynamics, including discrimination and poverty. Prevention success is not based on any one program, policy, or approach. It's about embedding new thinking and solutions into our organizations, literally *institution*alizing health and equity in policies, practices, and community norms. Actualizing these goals is within reach.

But it's not just about measurable success. At the end of the day, quality prevention has helped real people's lives, and it really is the personal impact that matters most. A few years ago, I met with advocates working to protect women from intimate-partner violence. We were discussing the impact that changing norms could have in reducing women's risk, and I described the tobacco laws as an example. People had said it was impossible to go against a big industry like tobacco, which had a controlling influence over social norms. "Larry, you're making a mistake that will harm your career," a colleague warned. "They've got all the money, all the power, all the connections. Watch the movies—all the sexy people smoke." It was true. At that time, they mostly didn't show people having sex in the movies; they showed satisfied people smoking in bed after having sex. Industry had created these alluring associations, but the new no-smoking laws changed people's way of thinking and behaving.

During a break in the meeting, one of the leaders, whom I greatly admired for her dedication and success in protecting women, pulled me aside. She told me that the minute she had heard about the smoking ban on airlines, she had added a stopover to an upcoming cross-country flight so she wouldn't have to go five hours without smoking. A week later, she thought, "What am I doing? Why do I so desperately need to change my plans for a cigarette—to maintain a habit that puts my health at such risk?" Without hesitation, she reinstated her nonstop flight and quit smoking then and there. "So you might have saved my life," she said. It made me feel proud that those laws had had such a positive, tangible effect on someone I so respect. I felt inspired to know prevention was making a real difference in people's lives.

GENIUSES PREVENT

In commemoration of the Prevention Institute's fifteen-year anniversary, we commissioned a beautiful, unique rocking bench made by wood-craft artist Rufus Blunk, who fashioned it from a 1,000-year-old rescued redwood tree. You can see its history in its wood—the flood 800 years ago, the fire 625 years ago. The redwood tree can grow over 300 feet tall and live for over 2,000 years—but it cannot stand alone. Beneath the surface of every redwood is a vast, intertwining root network connecting each tree to its neighbor. When the storms blow against the redwood, it is able to survive and continue to thrive because it relies upon the strength of the whole forest.

With an understanding of this principle, the Prevention Institute has spent almost twenty years promoting community-wide well-being and fairness, by recognizing that the quality of the systems binding us together profoundly impacts every one of us. We've been one of many planting seeds of aspiration and action. My goal with the organization has been to help spark broad, comprehensive efforts and participate in their development. Each victory reinforces fairness and wellness as optimal values and norms. As more stakeholders become invested, or are supported and listened to, our root system deepens.

Prevention is possible. As a country, we just have to stop getting in its way. Historically, when people and communities confront obstacles, every breakthrough is preceded by people shouting, "It's impossible!" As Nelson Mandela said, "It always seems impossible until it's done." Ultimately, it takes a critical mass of people thinking in a different way, promulgating a new approach, and advocating for the kind of community health where medicine is necessary but also the last resort. The issue is not just knowing what to do but getting it done. I call it political will, but really it's the common sense that comes from *all of us* demanding that our politicians, government, and corporations take actions to improve our communities as a way to advance health, not illness.

Albert Einstein said, "Intellectuals solve problems; geniuses prevent them." Everyone has a part to play in preventing health and safety problems and advancing equality in health and safety. It isn't just genius; together, we can, and we must, insist on health. And in the end we *will* create thriving, equitable, and safe communities.

As I was walking along the beach with my dog, a large flock of sandpipers swept along the shore. My dog saw them and gave chase. They took off easily and willingly. As they flew, they turned as one toward the sun in a way that created a silvery glint and made them seem to disappear. With one bird in the lead, effortlessly replaced by another, they flew in a V pattern—they looked almost like one body, responding to the cues of one another. It's not a coincidence that birds fly together. They carefully position their wingtips and sync their flapping to reduce each bird's use of energy—creating shared ease, resilience, and sustainable flight. It takes a flock to make a bird soar.

NOTES

Chapter 1

1. World Health Organization, Global Health Observatory Data Repository, Health expenditure ratios, all countries, selected years: Estimates by country. Retrieved from http://apps.who.int/gho/data/node.main.75

2. Olshansky, S. J., Passaro, D. J., Hershow, R. C., Layden, J. L., Carnes, B. A., Brody, J., . . . Ludwig, D. S. (2005). A potential decline in life expectancy in the United States in the 21st century. *The New England Journal of Medicine, 352,* 1138–1145. Retrieved from doi:10.1056/NEJMsr043743

3. Bipartisan Policy Center. (2012). Lots to lose: How America's health and obesity crisis threatens our economic future. Retrieved from http://bipartisanpolicy. org/library/lots-lose-how-americas-health-and-obesity-crisis-threatens-our-economic-future/

4. Ibid.

5. Lightwood, J., & Glantz, S.A. (2013). The effect of the California tobacco control program on smoking prevalence, cigarette consumption, and healthcare costs: 1989–2008. *PLoS One, 8*(2), e47145.

6. Cohen, L., & Swift, S. (1999). The spectrum of prevention: Developing a comprehensive approach to injury prevention. *Injury Prevention, 5*(3), 203–207.

7. Marmot, M., Friel, S., Bell, R., Houweling, T. A., Taylor, S., & Commission on Social Determinants of Health. (2008). Closing the gap in a generation: health equity through action on the social determinants of health. *The Lancet, 372*(9650), 1661–1669.

Chapter 2

1. Malins, J. (1936). A fence or an ambulance? In H. Feldman (Ed.), *The best loved poems of the American people*. Garden City, NY: Doubleday.
2. Steinem, G. (2002). Speech to the Commonwealth Club, San Francisco.
3. Rose, G., Khaw, K.-T., & Marmot, M. G. (2008). *Rose's strategy of preventive medicine: The complete original text* (2nd ed.). Oxford: Oxford University Press.
4. Robare, J. F. (2008). Prevention Research: The Center for Healthy Aging Demonstration Project. ProQuest.
5. Needleman, H. L. (1992). The current status of childhood low-level lead toxicity. *Neurotoxicology, 14*(2–3), 161–166.
6. Center for Disease Control and Prevention. (2014, September 12). Lead screening and prevalence of blood lead levels in children aged 1–2 Years: Child Blood Lead Surveillance System, United States, 2002–2010 and National Health and Nutrition Examination Survey, United States, 1999–2010. Retrieved from http://www.cdc.gov/mmwr/preview/mmwrhtml/su6302a6.htm
7. Gould, E. (2009). Childhood lead poisoning: Conservative estimates of the social and economic benefits of lead hazard control. *Environmental Health Perspectives, 117*(7), 1162–1167.
8. Birn, A.-E., & Brown, T. M. (Eds.). (2013). *Comrades in health: US health internationalists, abroad and at home*. New Brunswick, NJ: Rutgers University Press.
9. Henson, T. Jack Geiger, MD, M.Sc., ScD. (2014, March 10). Retrieved from http://wearepublichealthproject.org/interview/jack-geiger/
10. Ibid.

Chapter 3

1. Warner, K. E. (2006). *Tobacco control policy*, Vol. 21. New York: John Wiley.
2. Personal interview with M. Pertschuk (2016).
3. Hemenway, D. (2009). *While we were sleeping: Success stories in injury and violence prevention*. Berkeley: University of California Press.
4. Starnes, M. (2005). *Lives saved calculations for infants and toddlers*. Washington, DC: National Highway Traffic Safety Administration. Retrieved from http://www-nrd.nhtsa.dot.gov/Pubs/809778.pdf
5. Johnston, L. D. (2010). *Monitoring the future: National survey results on drug use, 1975–2008*, Vol. II: *College students and adults ages 19–50*. Bethesda, MD: National Institute on Drug Abuse.
6. Drunk driving fatalities drop below 10,000. (2016, January 6). Retrieved from http://www.madd.org/blog/2016/drunk-driving-fatalities-drop.html
7. Cohen, L., & Swift, S. (1999). The spectrum of prevention: Developing a comprehensive approach to injury prevention. *Injury Prevention, 5*, 203–207. Retrieved from http://www.odvn.org/training/Documents/doc-spectrum-prevention.pdf

8. Ibid.
9. Has, B. (2004). State-wide support for physician-mothers who are breastfeeding. *Work, 10,* 13–14.
10. Rodriguez-Garcia, R., & Frazier, L. (1995). Cultural paradoxes relating to sexuality and breastfeeding. *Journal of Human Lactation, 11*(2), 111–115.
11. Ryan, A. S., & Martinez, G. A. (1989). Breast-feeding and the working mother: A profile. *Pediatrics, 83*(4), 524–531.
12. Nguyen, T. T., & Hawkins, S. S. (2013). Current state of US breastfeeding laws. *Maternal & Child Nutrition, 9*(3), 350–358.

Chapter 4

1. UK Parliament. (n.d.). Churchill and the Commons Chamber. Retrieved from http://www.parliament.uk/about/living-heritage/building/palace/architecture/palacestructure/churchill/
2. Frank, L. D., Andresen, M. A., & Schmid, T. L. (2004). Obesity relationships with community design, physical activity, and time spent in cars. *American Journal of Preventive Medicine, 27*(2), 87–96.
3. Morland, K., Diez Roux, A. V., & Wing, S. (2006). Supermarkets, other food stores, and obesity: The Atherosclerosis Risk in Communities Study. *American Journal of Preventive Medicine, 30*(4), 333–339.
4. Change Lab Solutions. (2009). Establishing protections for community gardens: A fact sheet for advocates. Retrieved from http://www.changelabsolutions.org/sites/default/files/CommunityGarden_FactSht_21041106.pdf
5. DiMaggio, C., & Li, G. (2013). Effectiveness of a safe routes to school program in preventing school-aged pedestrian injury. *Pediatrics, 131*(2), 290–296.
6. Krieger, J., & Higgins, D. L. (2002). Housing and health: Time again for public health action. *American Journal of Public Health, 92*(5), 758–768.
7. Institute of Medicine. Committee on Assuring the Health of the Public in the 21st Century. (2003). *The future of the public's health in the 21st century.* Washington, DC: National Academy Press.
8. Associated Press. (2009, September 18). Parking spaces morph into "parks" across U.S.: Movement aims to "reimagine the possibilities of the urban landscape." Retrieved from http://www.nbcnews.com/id/32916362/ns/us_news-environment/t/parking-spaces-morph-parks-across-us/
9. Rebar Group, Inc. (2012). About Park(ing) Day. Retrieved from http://parkingday.org/about-parking-day/
10. Jaffe, D. (2014, June 14). Berkeley's first 2 parklets to open this fall. *Berkeleyside.* Retrieved from http://www.berkeleyside.com/2014/06/19/berkeleys-first-two-parklets-coming-this-fall/for
11. Loukaitou-Sideris, A., Brozen, M., Callahan, C. K., Brookover, I., LaMontagne, N., & Snehansh, V. (2012). *Reclaiming the right-of-way: A toolkit for creating and implementing parklets.* Los Angeles: Luskin Center for Innovation.

12. Cohen, D. A., Inagami, S., & Finch, B. (2008). The built environment and collective efficacy. *Health & Place, 14*(2), 198–208.

13. Exploratorium. (2015, March 17). New parklet adds informal science learning, STEM to Mission District. Press release. Retrieved from http://www.exploratorium.edu/press-office/press-releases/new-parklet-adds-informal-science-learning-stem-mission-district

14. Beveridge, C. (n.d.). *Frederick Law Olmsted Sr.: Landscape architect, author, conservationist (1822–1903)*. Washington, DC: National Association for Olmsted Parks. Retrieved from http://www.olmsted.org/the-olmsted-legacy/frederick-law-olmsted-sr

15. Frederick Law Olmsted. (2011). Olmsted's philosophy. Retrieved from http://www.fredericklawolmsted.com/philos.html

16. Fahim, K. (2010, April 5). Returning Prospect Park to the people. *The New York Times*. Retrieved from http://www.nytimes.com/2010/04/06/nyregion/06t upper.html?_r=0

17. Ibid.

18. Christoffel, T., & Gallagher, S. S. (2006). *Injury prevention and public health: Practical knowledge, skills, and strategies*. Burlington, MA: Jones & Bartlett Learning.

19. Prevention Institute. (2008, May). Strategies for enhancing the built environment to support healthy eating and active living. Retrieved from http://www.preventioninstitute.org/component/jlibrary/article/id-60/127.html

20. Frumkin, H., Frank, L., & Jackson, R. (2004). *Urban sprawl and public health*. Washington, DC: Island Press.

21. Prevention Institute, Strategies for enhancing the built environment.

22. Dannenberg, A. L., Frumkin, H., & Jackson, R. J. (2011). *Making healthy places*. Island Press, Washington, D.C.

23. Gauderman, W. J., et al. (2004). The effect of air pollution on lung development from 10 to 18 years of age. *The New England Journal of Medicine, 351*, 1057–1067. Retrieved from http://www.nejm.org/doi/full/10.1056/NEJMoa040610#t=abstract

24. American Planning Association. (2011). *Comprehensive planning for public health: Results of the Planning and Community Health Research Center Survey*. Retrieved from https://www.planning.org/research/publichealth/pdf/surveyreport.pdf

25. Fullilove, M. (2015). Fitcity 10 health keynote. Retrieved from https://vimeo.com/129237591

26. Fullilove, M. T., & Wallace, R. (2011). Serial forced displacement in American cities, 1916–2010. *Journal of Urban Health, 88*(3), 381–389.

27. International Making Cities Livable LLC. (2013). The other side of gentrification: Health effects of displacement. Retrieved from http://www.livablecities.org/blog/other-side-gentrification-health-effects-displacement

28. Fullilove & Wallace, Serial forced displacement in American cities.
29. Pyatok, M. (2005). The new urbanism: To whom should we listen? The social policies of urban renewal. *Newvillage*. Retrieved from http://www.newvillage. net/Journal/Issue2/2newurbanism.html
30. American Public Health Association & Urban Design 4 Health. (2010). The hidden health costs of transportation. Retrieved from https://www.apha.org/publications-and-periodicals/reports-and-issue-briefs/transportation
31. Cabanuatan, M. (2011, December 13). Bay Bridge bike path plans move forward. *SFGate*. Retrieved from http://www.sfgate.com/bayarea/article/Bay-Bridge-bike-path-plans-move-forward-2399824.php
32. American Public Health Association & Urban Design 4 Health, The hidden health costs of transportation.
33. Maus, J. (2011, October 13). Giant remakes GM ad and other reactions to the story. Retrieved from http://bikeportland.org/2011/10/13/giant-remakes-gm-ad-and-other-reactions-to-the-fiasco-60505
34. California Department of Transportation. (n.d.). Bicycle and pedestrian path. Retrieved from http://www.baybridgeinfo.org/path
35. Vanderbilt, T. (2011, July 15). Carmageddon challenge: Can Los Angeles cyclists beat a plane from Burbank to Long Beach? How my idle tweet spawned an epic transportation showdown. *Slate*. Retrieved from http://www.slate.com/articles/life/transport/2011/07/carmageddon_challenge.html
36. Ibid.
37. Active Transportation Alliance. (n.d.). About us. Retrieved from http://activetrans.org/
38. Pedestrians Educating Drivers on Safety. (n.d.). Report hazard facing people who walk. Retrieved from http://peds.org/
39. Fenway Alliance. (n.d.). Ten things we do: A summary of member benefits. Retrieved from http://fenwayculture.org/
40. Aboelata, M. J. (2004). *The built environment and health: 11 profiles of neighborhood transformation*. Oakland, CA: Prevention Institute.
41. Peñalosa, E. (2013, December 8). Enrique Peñalosa: Why buses represent democracy in action [Video]. Retrieved from http://www.ted.com/talks/enrique_penalosa_why_buses_represent_democracy_in_action
42. Gern, J. E., Reardon, C. L., Hoffjan, S., Nicolae, D., Li, Z., Roberg, K. A., . . . Lemanske, R. L. (2004). Effects of dog ownership and genotype on immune development and atopy in infancy. *Journal of Allergy and Clinical Immunology, 113*(2), 307–314.
43. Bergroth, E., Remes, S., Pekkanen, J., Kauppila, T., Büchele, G., & Keski-Nisula, L. (2012). Respiratory tract illnesses during the first year of life: Effect of dog and cat contacts. *Pediatrics, 130*(2), 1–10. Retrieved from doi:10.1542/peds.2011-2825

44. Daly, B., & Morton, L. (2006). An investigation of human–animal interactions and empathy as related to pet preference, ownership, attachment, and attitudes in children. *Anthrozoös, 19*(2), 113–127.
45. Bryant, B. (1990). The richness of the child–pet relationship: Consideration of both benefits and costs to children. *Anthrozoös, 3*(4), 253–261.
46. Banks, M., & Banks, W. (2002). The effects of animal-assisted therapy on loneliness in an elderly population in long-term care facilities. *The Journals of Gerontology: Series A, 57*(7), 428–432.
47. Le Roux, M., & Kemp, R. (2009). Effects of a companion dog on depression and anxiety levels of elderly residents in a long-term care facility. *Psychogeriatrics, 9*(1), 23–26.
48. Turner, W. (2007). The experiences of offenders in a prison canine program. *Federal Probation, 71*(1), 38–43.
49. Harkrader, T., Burke, T. W., & Owen, S. S. (2004). Pound puppies: The rehabilitative uses of dogs in correctional facilities. *Corrections Today, 66*(2), 74–79.
50. Britton, D., & Button, A. (2005). Prison pups: Assessing the effects of dog training programs in correctional facilities. *Journal of Family Social Work, 9*(4), 79–95.

Chapter 5

1. Collins, C., & Williams, D. (2001). Racial residential segregation: A fundamental cause of racial disparities in health. *Public Health Reports, 116*(5), 404–416.
2. Squires, G. D., & Kubrin, C. E. (2005). Privileged places: Race, uneven development and the geography of opportunity in urban America. *Urban Studies, 42*(1), 47–68.
3. Iton, T., Witt, S., & Kears, D. (2008). *Life and death from unnatural causes: Health and social inequity in Alameda County.* Oakland, CA: Alameda County Public Health Department.
4. Tavernise, S. (2011, October 24). Outside Cleveland, snapshots of poverty's surge in the suburbs. *The New York Times.*
5. World Health Organization. (2005). Interview with Professor Sir Michael Marmot. Retrieved from http://www.who.int/social_determinants/thecommission/marmot/en/
6. Foo, B. Two trains: Sonification of income inequality on the NYC subway's 2 train. Retrieved from https://vimeo.com/118358642.
7. Slaton, J. (2002, March 4). Oakland's toxic legacy; West Oakland pays the price for technological advancements. *San Francisco Chronicle.* Retrieved from http://www.sfgate.com/news/article/Oakland-s-Toxic-Legacy-West-Oakland-pays-the-2868916.php
8. Clay, E. A. (2016). Changing lives psychological research. *Monitor on Psychology, 47*(1), 34.

9. Kuo, F. E. (2001). Coping with poverty: Impacts of environment and attention in the inner city. *Environment and Behavior, 33*(1), 5–34.

10. Kuo, F. E., & Sullivan, W. C. (2001). Environment and crime in the inner city: Does vegetation reduce crime? *Environment and Behavior, 33*(3), 343–367.

11. Ibid.

12. Branas, C. C., Cheney, R. A., MacDonald, J. M., Tam, V. W., Jackson, T. D., & Ten Have, T. R. (2011). A difference-in-differences analysis of health, safety, and greening vacant urban space. *American Journal of Epidemiology, 174*(11), 1296–1306.

13. Cohen, L., Davis, R., & Parks, L. (2005, July). *Toward a lifetime commitment to violence prevention in Alameda County*. Oakland, CA: Prevention Institute.

14. The Godfather of sprawl. (1999, May 26). *The Atlantic Monthly*. Retrieved from https://www.theatlantic.com/past/docs/unbound/flashbks/moses.htm

15. Goldberger, P. (1981, July 30). Robert Moses, master builder, is dead at 92. *The New York Times*. Retrieved from http://www.nytimes.com/learning/general/onthisday/bday/1218.html

16. Moses, R. (1945, January). Slums and city planning. *The Atlantic*.

17. Bay Area Census. (n.d.). City of Oakland, Alameda County. Retrieved from http://www.bayareacensus.ca.gov/cities/Oakland70.htm

18. Badger, E. (2016, January 15). The inequality of sidewalks. *The Washington Post*. Retrieved from https://www.washingtonpost.com/news/wonk/wp/2016/01/15/the-inequality-of-sidewalks/

19. Personal interview with M. Gordon, 2011.

20. Ibid.

21. Pacific Institute for Studies in Development, Environment, and Security. (2002). Neighborhood knowledge for change: The West Oakland environmental indicators project. Retrieved from http://www.pacinst.org/wp-content/uploads/sites/21/2013/02/neighborhood_knowledge_for_change3.pdf

22. Slack G. (2002, February 20). Red Star's rising opposition. *East Bay Express*. Retrieved from www.mindfully.org/Air/Red-Star-West-Oakland20feb02.htm

23. Ibid.

24. Fleischer, D. Z., & Zames, F. (2001). *The disability rights movement: From charity to confrontation*. Philadelphia, PA: Temple University Press.

25. Personal interview with E. Roberts (1990).

26. Mattlin, B. (2012). *Miracle boy grows up: How the disability rights revolution saved my sanity*. New York: Skyhorse.

27. Geronimus, A. T., Hicken, M., Keene, D., & Bound, J. (2006). "Weathering" and age patterns of allostatic load scores among blacks and whites in the United States. *American Journal of Public Health, 96*(5), 826–833.

28. McEwen B. (1998). *Stress: How stress works*. Sydney: Australian Broadcasting Corporation.

29. City of Philadelphia Mural Arts Program: Philadelphia, PA. Retrieved from http://muralarts.org/
30. Millett, K. (1970). *Sexual politics*. Urbana: University of Illinois Press.
31. Courtenay, W. (2011). *Dying to be men: Psychosocial, environmental, and biobehavioral directions in promoting the health of men and boys*. New York: Routledge.
32. Durso, L. E., & Gates, G. J. (2012). Serving our youth: Findings from a national survey of service providers working with lesbian, gay, bisexual, and transgender youth who are homeless or at risk of becoming homeless. Los Angeles: The Williams Institute with True Colors Fund and The Palette Fund. Retrieved from http://williamsinstitute.law.ucla.edu/wp-content/uploads/Durso-Gates-LGBT-Homeless-Youth-Survey-July-2012.pdf
33. Kosciw, J. G., Greytak, E. A., Bartkiewicz, M. J., Boesen, M. J., & Palmer, N. A. (2012). *The 2011 National School Climate Survey: The experiences of lesbian, gay, bisexual and transgender youth in our nation's schools*. New York: GLSEN.
34. Ray, N. (2006). Lesbian, gay, bisexual and transgender youth: An epidemic of homelessness. New York: National Gay and Lesbian Task Force Policy Institute and the National Coalition for the Homeless. Retrieved from http://www.thetaskforce.org/static_html/downloads/HomelessYouth.pdf
35. Kelley, B. & Kelley S. (2011, September 1). Too pretty to do homework? [Web log post]. Huffington Post Retrieved from http://www.huffingtonpost.com/shannon-kelley/too-pretty-to-do-homework_b_944941.html
36. Occupy Wall Street is a people-powered movement that began in 2011 in New York City's Wall Street financial district, spawning the Occupy movement against social and economic inequality worldwide, with more than 100 participating US cities and actions in more than 1,500 cities globally. About Occupy Wall Street. (n.d.). Retrieved from http://occupywallst.org/about/
37. CBS & Time. (1999). *People of the century: One hundred men and women who shaped the last one hundred years*. New York: Simon & Schuster.
38. http://blacklivesmatter.com/guiding-principles/
39. Gaza, A. (n.d.). HerStory of the #BlackLivesMatter Movement. Retrieved from http://blacklivesmatter.com/herstory/
40. Ibid.

Chapter 6

1. Nestle, M. (2010). *What to eat*. New York: Macmillan.
2. Etherton, L., Russo, M., & Hossain, N. (2012). *Apples to Twinkies 2012: Comparing taxpayer subsidies for fresh produce and junk food*. Washington, DC: US PIRG. Retrieved from http://uspirg.org/sites/pirg/files/reports/Apples%20to%20Twinkies%20vUS_2.pdf
3. Reedy, J., & Krebs-Smith, S. M. (2010). Dietary sources of energy, solid fats, and added sugars among children and adolescents in the United States. *Journal of the American Dietetic Association, 110*(10), 1477–1484.

4. Ibid.
5. Centers for Disease Control and Prevention, US Department of Health and Human Services. (2008). *Physical activity and good nutrition: Essential elements to prevent chronic diseases and obesity*. Atlanta: Centers for Disease Control and Prevention.
6. Personal interview with B. Coleman (2001).
7. University of California, Los Angeles. (2012). Jonathan and Karin Fielding School of Public Health. Richard Joseph Jackson, M.D., M.P.H.
8. Watson, B.(2012, January 4). How the (finally ended) corn ethanol subsidy made us fatter. *Daily Finance*. Retrieved from http://www.dailyfinance.com/2012/01/04/how-the-finally-ended-corn-ethanol-subsidy-made-us-fatter/
9. California School Boards Association. (2015). Fact sheet: Drinking water access in schools. California Department of Public Health. https://www.csba.org/GovernanceAndPolicyResources/~/media/CSBA/Files/GovernanceResources/GovernanceBriefs/201504_DrinkingWaterAccessInSchools.ashx
10. Harris, J. L., Speers, S. E., Schwartz, M. B., & Brownell, K. B. (2012). US food company branded advergames on the Internet: Children's exposure and effects on snack consumption. *Journal of Children and Media, 6*(1), 51–68.
11. Mendoza, J. A., Zimmerman, F. J., & Christakis, D. A. (2007). Television viewing, computer use, obesity, and adiposity in U.S. preschool children. *The International Journal of Behavioral Nutrition and Physical Activity, 4*, 44.
12. Mikkelsen, L., Merlo, C., Lee, V., & Chao, C. (2007). *Where's the fruit? Fruit content of the most highly-advertised children's food and beverages*. Oakland, CA: Prevention Institute. Retrieved from http://www.preventioninstitute.org/component/jlibrary/article/id-56/127.html
13. Sims, J., Mikkelsen, L., Gibson, P., & Warming, E. (2010). *Claiming health: Front-of-package labeling of children's food*. Oakland, CA: Prevention Institute. Retrieved from http://www.preventioninstitute.org/component/jlibrary/article/id-293/127.html
14. MSNBC. (2007). How much fruit is in fruit juice? *The Today Show*.
15. US Department of Agriculture. (n.d.). National School Lunch Program. Retrieved from http://www.fns.usda.gov/nslp/national-school-lunch-program-nslp
16. Johnson, D. B., Podrabsky, M., Rocha, A., & Otten, J. J. (2016). Effect of the Healthy Hunger-Free Kids Act on the nutritional quality of meals selected by students and school lunch participation rates. *JAMA Pediatrics, 170*(1), e153918–e153918.
17. Edible East Bay. (2015, November 16). A tale of two West Oakland farms. Retrieved from http://edibleeastbay.com/online-magazine/winter-holidays-2015/a-tale-of-two-west-oakland-farms/
18. Stanford Report. (2010). *New report reveals the environmental and social impact of the "livestock revolution."* Stanford University News: Stanford Universtiy.
19. Vegetarismus.com. (2012, November 13). SVV: The ecological consequences of meat consumption. Retrieved from http://www.vegetarismus.com/info/eoeko.htm

20. United States Department of Agriculture. (2013). Data pulled from The ERS Food Availability (Per Capita) Data System (FADS). Retrieved from http://www.ers.usda.gov/data-products/food-availability-%28per-capita%29-data-system/summary-findings.aspx

21. World Cancer Research Fund / American Institute for Cancer Research. (2007). *Food, nutrition, physical activity, and the prevention of cancer: A global perspective.* Retrieved from http://www.wcrf.org/sites/default/files/Second-Expert-Report.pdf

22. The International Agency for Research on Cancer. (2015). IARC Monographs evaluate consumption of red meat and processed meat. [Press release]. Retrieved from https://www.google.com/url?sa=t&rct=j&q=&esrc=s&source=web&cd=1&cad=rja&uact=8&ved=0ahUKEwi1sL_n3b7KAhUBzmMKHfpeB-gQFggdMAA&url=https%3A%2F%2Fwww.iarc.fr%2Fen%2Fmedia-centre%2Fpr%2F2015%2Fpdfs%2Fpr240_E.pdf&usg=AFQjCNHKyMQoMO-GMCpD5vb35LnmNtsMPg&sig2=_TgTbrHgaJQTOLgQsQIqRg

23. US Department of Agriculture, Economic and Research Service. (2016). Ag and food sectors and the economy. Retrieved from http://www.ers.usda.gov/data-products/ag-and-food-statistics-charting-the-essentials/ag-and-food-sectors-and-the-economy.aspx

24. Ringgenberg, W. J. W. (2014). Trends and characteristics of occupational suicide and homicide in farmers and agriculture workers, 1992–2010. Ph.D. diss., University of Iowa, Iowa City. Retrieved from http://ir.uiowa.edu/etd/4734/

25. Bureau of Labor Statistics. (2015). Occupational employment statistics. Retrieved from http://www.bls.gov/oes/current/oes_nat.htm

26. Government Accountability Office. (2005, January) Workplace safety and health. Retrieved from http://www.gao.gov/new.items/d0596.pdf

27. National Institute for Occupational Safety and Health. (n.d.) Agricultural safety. Retrieved from http://www.cdc.gov/niosh/topics/aginjury/

28. US Department of Health and Human Services, Administration of Children and Families, Office of Community Services. (n.d.). Healthy food financing initiative. Retrieved from http://www.acf.hhs.gov/programs/ocs/programs/community-economic-development/healthy-food-financing

29. Dimitri, C., & Greene, C. (2002). Recent growth patterns in the US organic foods market. Agriculture Information Bulletin 777. Retrieved from http://www.ers.usda.gov/publications/aib-agricultural-information-bulletin/aib777.aspx

30. Food Research and Action Center. (2012). A review of strategies to bolster SNAP's role in improving nutrition as well as food security. Retrieved from http://frac.org/wp-content/uploads/2011/06/SNAPstrategies.pdf

31. Marin, P., Vaupel, S., Amaya, W., Fish, C., & Amon, R. (1985). The fragmented California farm labor market. *California Agriculture, 39*(11), 14–16.

32. Food Trust. (2004).Pennsylvania Fresh Food Financing Initiative. Retrieved from http://thefoodtrust.org/uploads/media_items/hffi-one-pager.original.pdf

33. Food Trust. (2004). The Food Trust Mission: Ensuring that everyone has access to affordable, nutritious food. Retrieved from http://thefoodtrust.org

34. Agricultural Act of 2014, H.R. 2642, 2nd Cong. (2014).

35. Lee, H., & Sumner, D. A. (2014). The 2014 Farm Bill, commodity subsidies, and California agriculture. *Agricultural and Resource Economics Update*, 17(4),1–4. Retrieved from http://giannini.ucop.edu/media/are-update/files/issues/V17N4_1.pdf

36. Ibid.

37. Imhoff, D. (2012, March 21). Overhauling the Farm Bill: The real beneficiaries of subsidies. *The Atlantic.* Retrieved from http://www.theatlantic.com/health/archive/2012/03/overhauling-the-farm-bill-the-real-beneficiaries-of-subsidies/254422/

38. Smith R. (2011, July 29). Rural population decline poses ag program challenges. *Farm Press.* Retrieved from http://deltafarmpress.com/blog/rural-population-decline-poses-ag-program-challenges

39. Food and Agriculture Policy Collaborative. (n.d.). Healthy food, healthy economies. Retrieved from http://frac.org/pdf/food_ag_policy_collaborative_hfhe.pdf

40. Krueger, J. E., Krub, K. R., & Hayes, L. A. (2010). *Planting the seeds for public health: How the Farm Bill can help farmers to produce and distribute healthy foods.* St. Paul, MN: Farmers Legal Action Group.

41. Billings, D. & Markowitz, L.(2010). Kentucky's Community Farm Alliance: From growing tobacco to building the good L.I.F.E. Solutions for a sustainable and desirable future. 1(4).

42. Ibid.

43. Community Farm Alliance. (n.d.). *History: A chronicle of successful organizing.* Retrieved from http://cfaky.org/aboutcfa/history/

44. Small, S. (2015, August 8). Stronger together: How Community Farm Alliance supports Kentucky's farming community. *Food Tank.* Retrieved from http://farmdocdaily.illinois.edu/2014/02/evaluating-commodity-program-choices-in-new-farm-bill.html

45. US Department of Agriculture. (2014). Food away from home. Retrieved from http://www.ers.usda.gov/topics/food-choices-health/food-consumption-demand/food-away-from-home.aspx

46. California Center for Public Health Advocacy.(2012). Legislative successes. Retrieved from http://www.publichealthadvocacy.org/legislation.html

47. Taber, D. R., Chriqui, J. F., & Chaloupka, F. J. (2012). Differences in nutrient intake associated with state laws regarding fat, sugar, and caloric content of competitive foods. *Archives of Pediatrics & Adolescent Medicine, 166*(5), 452–458.

Chapter 7

1. Centers for Disease Control and Prevention. (2013). 10 leading causes of death by age group, United States. Retrieved from http://www.cdc.gov/injury/images/lc-charts/leading_causes_of_death_by_age_group_2013-a.gif

2. Centers for Disease Control and Prevention. (2016). Cost of injuries and violence in the United States. Retrieved from http://www.cdc.gov/injury/wisqars/overview/cost_of_injury.html

3. Chandran, A., Hyder, A. A., & Peek-Asa, C. (2010). The global burden of unintentional injuries and an agenda for progress. *Epidemiologic Reviews,* *32*(1), 110–120.

4. Centers for Disease Control and Prevention. (n.d.). Emergency department visits. Retrieved from http://www.cdc.gov/nchs/fastats/emergency-department.htm

5. National Hospital Ambulatory Medical Care Survey: 2011 emergency department summary tables. (n.d.). Retrieved from http://www.cdc.gov/nchs/data/ahcd/nhamcs_emergency/2011_ed_web_tables.pdf

6. Centers for Disease Control and Prevention, National Center for Injury Prevention and Control, WISQARS. (2014). Leading causes of death reports, national and regional, 1999–2014. Retrieved from http://webappa.cdc.gov/sasweb/ncipc/leadcaus10_us.html

7. Centers for Disease Control and Prevention. (1999). Ten great public health achievements—United States, 1900–1999. *Morbidity and Mortality Weekly Report, 48*(12), 241.

8. Jones, B., Dellinger, A., & Wallace, D. (1999). Achievements in public health, 1900–1999. Motor vehicle safety: A 20th century public health achievement. *Morbidity and Mortality Weekly Report, 48,* 369–374.

9. Children's Safety Network. (2005). *Child safety seats: How large are the benefits and who should pay?* Calverton, MD: Children's Safety Network Economics and Data Analysis Resource Center.

10. Kaiser Permanente. (2012, February 20). The president, the first lady, and Henry J. Kaiser. Retrieved from http://kaiserpermanentehistory.org/latest/the-president-the-first-lady-and-henry-j-kaiser/

11. Kaiser Permanente. (2009, September 4). Richmond shipyard workers suffered their own casualties of war. Retrieved from https://kaiserpermanentehistory.org/latest/richmond-shipyard-workers-suffered-their-own-casualties-of-war/

12. Kaiser Permanente, The president, the first lady, and Henry J. Kaiser.

13. Kaiser Permanente, Richmond shipyard workers.

14. Marsh, S. M., Menendez, C. C., Baron, S. L., Steege, A. L., & Myers, J. R. (2013). Fatal work-related injuries—United States, 2005–2009. *Morbidity and Mortality Weekly Report, 62*(Suppl. 3), 41–45. http://www.cdc.gov/mmwr/preview/mmwrhtml/su6203a7.htm#Tab1

15. Byler, C. G. (2013). Hispanic/Latino fatal occupational injury rates. *Monthly Labor Review, 136*(2), 14–23.

16. Centers for Disease Control and Prevention. (n.d.). Benefits of health promotion programs. Retrieved from http://www.cdc.gov/workplacehealthpromotion/businesscase/benefits/

17. Centers for Medicare and Medicaid. (2014). National health expenditures 2014. Retrieved from https://www.cms.gov/Research-Statistics-Data-and-Systems/Statistics-Trends-and-Reports/NationalHealthExpendData/downloads/highlights.pdf

18. Baicker, K., Cutler, D., & Song, Z. (2010). Workplace wellness programs can generate savings. *Health Affairs, 29*(2), 304–311.

19. Committee on Injury and Poison Prevention. (2001). Falls from heights: Windows, roofs, and balconies. *Pediatrics, 107*(5), 1188–1191.

20. Barlow, B., Niemirska, M., Gandhi, R. P., & Leblanc, W. (1983). Ten years of experience with falls from a height in children. *Journal of Pediatric Surgery, 18*(4), 509–511.

21. Berg, R. L., & Cassells, J. S. (1990). *The second fifty years: Promoting health and preventing disability.* Washington, DC: National Academy Press.

22. Centers for Disease Control and Prevention. (n.d.) Costs of falls among older adults. Retrieved from http://www.cdc.gov/homeandrecreationalsafety/falls/fallcost.html

23. Administration on Aging. (n.d.). Projected future growth of the older population. Retrieved from http://www.aoa.acl.gov/aging_statistics/future_growth/future_growth.aspx#age

24. Carande-Kulis, V., Stevens, J. A., Florence, C. S., Beattie, B. L., & Arias, I. (2015). A cost–benefit analysis of three older adult fall prevention interventions. *Journal of Safety Research, 52*, 65–70.

25. Illinois Poison Center. (2011). These darn safety caps are a pain in the.... Retrieved from http://ipcblog.org/2011/03/22/%E2%80%9Cthese-darn-safety-caps-are-a-pain-in-the%E2%80%A6%E2%80%9D/

26. Kirk, N. S. (1981). Poison Prevention Packaging Act, 1970: A human factors standard. *Applied Ergonomics, 12*(4), 195–201.

27. Centers for Disease Control and Prevention. (2013). 10 leading causes of injury deaths by age group highlighting unintentional injury deaths, United States: 2013. Retrieved from http://www.cdc.gov/injury/images/lc-charts/leading_causes_of_injury_deaths_highlighting_unintentional_injury_2013-a.gif

28. National SAFE KIDS Campaign. (2004). *Children at risk fact sheet.* Washington, DC: National Center for Children in Poverty.

29. Kreisberg, J. (2014, July 11). Alameda County Safe Medication Disposal Initiative Assessment. Teleosis Institute. Retrieved from http://www.teleosis.org/wp-content/uploads/2012/02/AlamedaCo_SafeMedDisposal_Assessment-Final_l.pdf

30. Ibid.
31. Hemenway, D. (2009). *While we were sleeping: Success stories in injury and violence prevention.* Berkeley. University of California Press.
32. About the Green Science Policy Institute. (n.d.). Retrieved from http://greensciencepolicy.org/about/
33. McGuire, A.(1999). How the tobacco industry continues to keep the home fires burning. *Tobacco Contro, 8*(1), 67–69.
34. Public Broadcasting Service. (n.d.). Anatomy of a cigarette. Retrieved from http://www.pbs.org/wgbh/nova/cigarette/anat_flash.html
35. McGuire, How the tobacco industry continues.
36. Taylor, M. (2015, February). The 2015-2016 Budget: Analysis of the Human Services Budget. Retrived from http://www.lao.ca.gov/reports/2015/budget/human-services/hs-analysis-021215.pdf
37. Thompson, D. C., & Rivara, F. P. (1998). Pool fencing for preventing drowning in children. *Cochrane Database of Systematic Reviews, 1.*
38. Merriam-Webster. (2012). Keiki. *Merriam-Webster Dictionary.*
39. Ocean Safety and Lifeguard Services Division of the City and County of Honolulu's Emergency Services Department. (2005). Ocean Safety & Lifeguard Services. Retrieved from http://www.honolulu.gov/esdosls.html
40. Luo M. (2004, February 27). For exercise in New York futility, push button. *The New York Times.* Retrieved from http://www.nytimes.com/2004/02/27/nyregion/for-exercise-in-new-york-futility-push-button.html?_r=0
41. Ibid.
42. Bechtel, A. K., MacLeod, K. E., & Ragland, D. R. (2003). Oakland Chinatown pedestrian scramble: An evaluation. Retrieved from http://escholarship.org/uc/item/3fh5q4dk
43. Kattan, L., Acharjee, S., & Tay, R. (2009). Pedestrian scramble operations. *Transportation Research Record: Journal of the Transportation Research Board, 2140,* 79–84.
44. O'Neil, B. (2002, January/February). Accidents or crashes: Highway safety and William Haddon Jr. *Contingencies,* 30–32.
45. Ibid.
46. Cohen, L. (2011, October 2). For want of a crosswalk, a life was lost. *The Huffington Post.* Retrieved from http://www.huffingtonpost.com/larry/for-want-of-a-crosswalk-a_b_913582.html
47. Ibid.
48. Ibid.
49. Georgia Department of Transportation. (2011). Amended FY 2010 & FY 2011 budget.
50. Centers for Disease Control and Prevention. (n.d.). Pedestrian safety. Retrieved from http://www.cdc.gov/motorvehiclesafety/pedestrian_safety/

51. America Bikes. (2012). National poll: Americans support funding for sidewalks and bikeways. Retrieved from http://www.bikeleague.org/sites/default/files/America_Bikes_White_paper_final.pdf
52. Fukushima, A. (2012). Caltrans embraces complete streets on the Central Coast. *Focus: Journal of the City and Regional Planning Department, 9*(1), 12.
53. Pucher, J., & Renne, J. L. (2003). Socioeconomics of urban travel: Evidence from the 2001 NHTS. *Transport Quarterly, 57*, 49.

Chapter 8

1. Centers for Disease Control and Prevention. (2014). Preventing youth violence: Opportunities for action. Retrieved from http://www.cdc.gov/violenceprevention/youthviolence/pdf/opportunities-for-action.pdf.
2. Center for Disease Control and Prevention. (2013). 10 leading causes of injury deaths by age group highlighting violence-related injury death, United States. Retrieved from http://www.cdc.gov/injury/wisqars/pdf/leading_causes_of_injury_death_highlighting_violence_2013-a.pdf
3. The Brady Campaign. (2015). Gun death injury stat sheet 5-year average. Retrieved from http://www.bradycampaign.org/sites/default/files/Gun-Death-Injury-Stat-Sheet-5-Year-Average-2013-Updates-Jan-2015.pdf
4. Children's Defense Fund. (2012). *Protect children, not guns.* Washington, DC: Children's Defense Fund.
5. Masters, M. (2016, January 12). U.S. gun policy: Global comparisons. Council on Foreign Relations. Retrieved from http://www.cfr.org/society-and-culture/us-gun-policy-global-comparisons/p29735
6. City of Minneapolis Health Department. (2013, August). Minneapolis Blueprint for Action to Prevent Youth Violence. Retrieved from http://www.minneapolismn.gov/www/groups/public/@health/documents/webcontent/wcms1p-121861.pdf
7. Prevention Institute. (2012, January). Public health contributions to preventing violence fact sheet. Retrieved from http://www.preventioninstitute.org/component/jlibrary/article/id-321/127.html
8. Lisak, D., & Beszterczey, S. (2007). The cycle of violence: The life histories of 43 death row inmates. *Psychology of Men & Masculinity, 8*(2), 118–128.
9. Smith, J. C. (Ed.). (1996). *Notable black American women*, Book II. Detroit: Gale.
10. Henrichson, C., & Delaney, R. (2012). The price of prisons: What incarcerations cost taxpayers. Vera Institute of Justice. Retrieved from http://www.vera.org/sites/default/files/resources/downloads/price-of-prisons-updated-version-021914.pdf
11. Centers for Disease Control and Prevention. (2012). Health, United States, 2012: With special feature on emergency care. Retrieved from http://www.cdc.gov/nchs/data/hus/hus12.pdf.

12. Vera Institute of Justice. (2012). The price of prisons: What incarceration costs taxpayers. Retrieved from http://www.vera.org/sites/default/files/resources/downloads/Price_of_Prisons_updated_version_072512.pdf

13. Stith, D. P. (1991). *Deadly consequences: How violence is destroying our teenage population and a plan to begin solving the problem.* New York: HarperCollins.

14. Earls, F. (1994). Violence and today's youth. *Critical Health Issues for Children and Youth,* 4(3). Retrieved from https://www.princeton.edu/futureofchildren/publications/journals/article/index.xml?journalid=61&articleid=384&sectionid=2593

15. Centers for Disease Control and Prevention. (2012, April 19). Protect the ones you love: Child injuries are preventable. Retrieved from http://www.cdc.gov/safechild/NAP/background.html

16. City-Data. (2013). Crime rate in Los Angeles, California (CA): Murders, rapes, robberies, assaults, burglaries, thefts, auto thefts, arson, law enforcement employees, police officers, crime map. Retrieved from http://www.city-data.com/crime/crime-Los-Angeles-California.html

17. Centers for Disease Control and Prevention. (2012). Youth violence: Facts at a glance. Retrieved from http://www.cdc.gov/violenceprevention/pdf/yv-datasheet-a.pdf

18. Dorfman, L., & Wallack, L. (2009). Moving from them to us: Challenges in reframing violence among youth. Retrieved from http://www.bmsg.org/resources/publications/moving-from-them-to-us-challenges-in-reframing-violence-among-youth

19. Dorfman, L. & Wallack, L. (2009). *Moving from them to us: Challenges in reframing violence among youth.* Retrieved from http://www.bmsg.org/pdfs/BMSGReframingViolenceRev.pdf

20. Cohen, L., Davis, R., Lee, V., & Valdovinos, E. (2010, May). Addressing the intersection: Preventing violence and promoting healthy eating and active living. Retrieved from http://www.preventioninstitute.org/component/jlibrary/article/id-267/127.html

21. Prevention Institute. (2011, May). Fact sheets: Links between violence and chronic diseases, mental illness and poor learning. Retrieved from http://www.preventioninstitute.org/component/jlibrary/article/id-301/127.html

22. Garcetti, G. (2011, March 25). Observations and provocations from the *Times'* opinion staff. Retrieved from http://opinion.latimes.com/opinionla/2011/03/gil-garcetti-californias-death-penalty-doesnt-serve-justice.html

23. Pitney, N. (2015, September 24). Nothing stops a bullet like a job. *The Huffington Post.* Retrieved from http://www.huffingtonpost.com/entry/greg-boyle-homeboy-industries-life-lessons_56030036e4b00310edf9c7a4

24. Ibid.

25. Why we do it. (n.d.) Retrieved from http://www.homeboyindustries.org/why-we-do-it/
26. Personal interview with F. Smith (2003)..
27. Designing Healthy Communities. (2010, October 4). Residents for safer, pedestrian-friendly environments. Retrieved from http://designinghealthycommunities.org/residents-safer-pedestrian-friendly-environment/.
28. Ruppert, B. (2014). The Statue of George III. *Journal of the American Revolution.* Retrieved from http://allthingsliberty.com/2014/09/the-statue-of-george-iii/
29. Personal interview with B. Weiss (2003).
30. Bureau of Justice Statistics. (1995, August). Violence against women: Estimates form the redesigned survey. Retrieved from http://www.bjs.gov/content/pub/pdf/FEMVIED.PDF
31. Fisher, B. S., Krebs, C. P., Lindquist, C. H., Martin, S. L., & Warner, T. D. (2009). College women's experiences with physically forced, alcohol- or other drug-enabled, and drug-facilitated sexual assault before and since entering college. *Journal of American College Health,* 57(6), 639–647.
32. Morgan, R. E., & Truman, J. L. (2014, April 16). Nonfatal domestic violence 2003–2012. Retrieved from http://www.bjs.gov/index.cfm?ty=pbdetail&iid=4985
33. Basile, K. C., Black, M. C., Breiding, M. J., Chen, J., Merrick, M. T., Smith, S. G., & Walters, M. L. (2011). *National Intimate Partner and Sexual Violence Survey: 2010 Summary Report.* Atlanta: Centers for Disease Control and Prevention, National Center for Injury Prevention and Control, Division of Violence Prevention.
34. Cohen, L. (2012). Larry Cohen's written testimony for the task force for defending childhood. Retrieved from http://www.preventioninstitute.org/about-us/lp/856-lc-testimony.html
35. The Associated Press. (1984, February 1). Update: Invaders' message is disturbing to Oakland. *The New York Times,* Retrieved from http://www.nytimes.com/
36. News Sentinel. (1984, February 1). Criticized Invaders ads "violent." Retrieved from https://news.google.com/newspapers?nid=2245&dat=19840201&id=7JUzAAAAIBAJ&sjid=bjIHAAAAIBAJ&pg=2848,3195491&hl=en
37. Desilver, D. (2013, June 4). A minority of Americans own guns, but just how many is unclear. Retrieved from http://www.pewresearch.org/fact-tank/2013/06/04/a-minority-of-americans-own-guns-but-just-how-many-is-unclear/
38. Prothrow-Stith, D., & Spivak, H. (2004). *Murder is no accident: Understanding and preventing youth violence in America.* San Francisco: Jossey-Bass.
39. Graduate Institute. (2009). Small arms survey 2009: Shadows of war. Retrieved from http://www.smallarmssurvey.org/fileadmin/docs/A-Yearbook/2009/en/Small-Arms-Survey-2009-Prelims-Intro-EN.pdf

40. Clark, V. Ruback, B., & Shaffer, J. (2011). Easy access to firearms: Juveniles' risks for violent offending and violent victimization. *Journal of Interpersonal Violence, 26*(10), 2111–2138.
41. Wilkinson, R., & Pickett, K. (2009). *The spirit level: Why greater equality makes societies stronger.* New York: Bloomsbury Press.
42. Center for the Study and Prevention of Violence. (n.d.). Facts. Retrieved from http://www.colorado.edu/cspv/
43. Associated Press. (2002, April 28). Bush owed presidency to NRA, NRA says. *Los Angeles Times.* Retrieved from http://articles.latimes.com/2002/apr/28/news/mn-40519.
44. Loujan, M (2011, January 25). NRA stymies firearms research, scientists say. *The New York Times.* Retrieved from http://www.nytimes.com/2011/01/26/us/26guns.html?_r=1
45. Shumaker, E. (2015, December 7). Why the ban on gun violence research is a public health issue. *The Huffington Post.* Retrieved from http://www.huffingtonpost.com/entry/dickey-amendment-gun-violence-research-ban_56606201e4b072e9d1c4eaaa
46. Dickey, J., & Rosenberg, M. (2010, July 27). We won't know the cause of gun violence until we look for it. *The Washington Post.* Retrieved from https://www.washingtonpost.com/opinions/we-wont-know-the-cause-of-gun-violence-until-we-look-for-it/2012/07/27/gJQAPfenEX_print.html
47. Inskeep, S. (2015). Ex-Rep. Dickey regrets restrictive law on gun violence research. NPR. Retrieved from http://www.npr.org/2015/10/09/447098666/ex-rep-dickey-regrets-restrictive-law-on-gun-violence-research.
48. US Supreme Court. (2007). *District of Columbia et al. v. Heller.* Retrieved from http://www.scotusblog.com/wp-content/uploads/2008/06/07- 290.pdf
49. Wiser, M. (Dir.). (2015). Gunned down: The power of the NRA. In M. Kirk, J. Gilmore, & M. Wiser (Prods.), *Frontline.* Boston: WGBH/Boston.
50. PACT. (n.d.). Taking aim at gun dealers: Contra Costa's public health approach to reducing firearms in the community. Retrieved from http://cchealth.org/topics/violence/pdf/taking_aim_at_gun_dealers.pdf
51. Cure Violence. (2014). Annual report 2014. Retrieved from http://cureviolence.org/wp-content/uploads/2015/06/Cure-Violence-Annual-Report-2014.pdf
52. Anda, R. F., Edwards, V., Felitti, V. J., Koss, M. P., Marks, J. S., Nordenberg, D., . . . Williamson, D. F. (1998). Relationship of childhood abuse and household dysfunction to many of the leading causes of death in adults. The Adverse Childhood Experiences (ACE) Study. *American Journal of Prevention Medicine, 14*(4), 245–258.
53. Anda, R. F., Chapman, D. F., Dong, M., Dube, S. R., Edwards, V. J., & Felitti, V. J. (2005). The wide-ranging health consequences of adverse childhood

experiences. *Victimization of children and youth: Patterns of abuse, response strategies.* New Jersey: Civic Research Institute.

54. Cohen, L., Davis, R., & Parks, L. (2005, July). *Toward a lifetime commitment to violence prevention in Alameda County.* Oakland, CA: Prevention Institute.

55. Prevention Institute. (2001, September). Preventing and reducing school violence fact sheets: What factors foster resiliency against violence? Retrieved from http://www.preventioninstitute.org/component/jlibrary/article/id-50/288.html

56. Felitti, V. J., Anda, R. F., Nordenberg, D., Williamson, D. F., Spitz, A. M., Edwards, V. E. . . . Marks, J. S. (1998). Relationship of childhood abuse and household dysfunction to many of the leading causes of death in adults: The Adverse Childhood Experiences (ACE) study. *American Journal of Preventive Medicine, 14*(4), 245–258.

57. Department of Education Office of Civil Rights. (2012). Civil rights data collection. Retrieved from http://ocrdata.ed.gov/

58. Teasley, M. (2004). Absenteeism and truancy: Risk, protection, and best practice implications for school social workers. *Children & Schools, 26*(2), 117–128.

59. L.A. schools will no longer suspend a student for being defiant. (2013, May 15). *Los Angeles Times.* Retrieved from http://articles.latimes.com/2013/may/15/local/la-me-ln-lausd-suspensions-20130515

60. Davis, R., & Pinderhughes, H. (2013, April). Addressing and preventing trauma at the community level. Retrieved from http://www.preventioninstitute.org/component/jlibrary/article/id-347/127.html

61. Weiss, B. (2008, June). An Assessment of Youth Violence Prevention Activities in USA Cities. Retrieved http://www.eatbettermovemore.org/documents/UNITY-SCIPRCassessmentJune2008pdfSECURED.pdf

62. Prevention Institute. (2008). Overview of the UNITY RoadMap: A Framework for Effective and Sustainable Efforts. Retrieved from http://www.preventioninstitute.org/index.php?option=com_jlibrary&view=article&id=30&Itemid=127

63. Branas, C. C., Cheney, R. A., MacDonald, J. M., Tam, V. W., Jackson, T. D., & Ten Have, T. R. (2011). A difference-in-differences analysis of health, safety, and greening vacant. *American Journal of Epidemiology, 171*(11), 1296-1306

64. City of Minneapolis Health Department. (2013, August). Minneapolis Blueprint for Action to Prevent Youth Violence. Retrieved from http://www.minneapolismn.gov/www/groups/public/@health/documents/webcontent/wcms1p-121861.pdf

65. Prevention Institute. (2010). A major milestone in preventing violence. [Press release]. Retrieved from http://www.preventioninstitute.org/press/press-releases/389-a-major-milestone-in-preventing-violence.html

66. Cohn, D., Taylor, P., Lopez, M. H., Gallagher, C. A., Parker, K. & Maass, K. T. (2013, May 7). Gun homicide rate down 49% since 1993 peak; public unaware. Retrieved from http://www.pewsocialtrends.org/2013/05/07/gun-homicide-rate-down-49-since-1993-peak-public-unaware/

67. Redburn, S., Travis, J., & Western, B. (2014). *The growth of incarceration in the United States: Exploring causes and consequences.* Washington, DC: National Academies Press.

68. California Department of Education. (2013). Current expense of education & per-pupil spending. Retrieved from http://www.cde.ca.gov/ds/fd/ec/currentexpense.asp

69. Demographic patterns of cumulative arrest prevalence by ages 18 and 23 (2014). *Crime & Delinquency, 60,* 471–486.

70. Wildeman, C. (2009). Parental imprisonment, the prison boom, and the concentration of childhood disadvantage. *Demography, 46*(2), 265–280.

71. Policy Link. (n.d.). Why place and race matter: Impacting health through a focus of place and race. Retrieved from http://www.policylink.org/sites/default/files/WHY_PLACE_AND_RACE%20MATTER_FULL%20REPORT_WEB.PDF

72. Pinderhughes, H., Davis, R., & Williams, M. (2016). Adverse community experiences and resilience. Retrieved from http://www.preventioninstitute.org/component/jlibrary/article/id-372/127.html

73. Dahlberg, L. (1998). Youth violence in the United States. Major trends, risk factors, and prevention approaches. *American Journal of Preventative Medicine, 14*(4), 259–272.

74. Cohen, L., & Swift, S. (1991). Beyond brochures: Preventing alcohol-related violence and injuries. Retrieved from http://thrive.preventioninstitute.org/alcohol.html.

75. Aboelata, M. (2004, July). The built environment and health: 11 profiles of neighborhood transformation. Retrieved from http://preventioninstitute.org

76. Themba-Nixon, M. (2010). The power of local communities to foster policy. In L. Cohen, S. Chehimi, & V. Chavez (Eds.), *Prevention is primary: Strategies for community well being* (2nd ed., pp. 137–156). San Francisco: Jossey-Bass.

77. Dahlberg, L. L., Krug, E. G., Lozano, R., Mercy, J. A., & Zwi, A. B. (2002). World report on violence and health. World Health Organization. Retrieved from http://www.who.int/violence_injury_prevention/violence/world_report/en/introduction.pdf

78. Ibid.

79. Chautauqua Institution. (2012, July 11). Krista Tippett with Father Greg Boyle on turning inspiration into action [Video]. Retrieved from https://www.youtube.com/watch?v=S9MkHqIMBfc

80. The Eleanor Roosevelt Papers Project. (n.d.). Quotations by Eleanor Roosevelt. Retrieved from https://www.gwu.edu/~erpapers/abouteleanor/er-quotes/

Chapter 9

1. Johnston, L., & Herman, R. (1983, February 28). New York day by day. *The New York Times*. Retrieved from http://www.nytimes.com/1983/02/28/nyregion/new-york-day-by-day-260701.html

2. Smith, E. A., & Malone, R. E. (2009). "Everywhere the soldier will be": Wartime tobacco promotion in the US military. *American Journal of Public Health, 99*(9), 1595–1602. Retrieved from http://doi.org/10.2105/AJPH.2008.152983

3. Hale, J. (1986, May 15). Prevent children from starting, anti-smoking. *Bangor Daily News*. Retrieved from http://news.google.com/newspapers?nid=2457&dat=19860514&id=Vo1eAAAAIBAJ&sjid=-E4NAAAAIBAJ&pg=6349,4781248

4. Garber, M. (2015, June 15). "You've come a long way, baby": The lag between advertising and feminism. *The Atlantic*. Retrieved from http://www.theatlantic.com/entertainment/archive/2015/06/advertising-1970s-womens-movement/395897/

5. Carpenter, D. (1987). "Emphysema slims": Doctors attack smoking with ridicule. *Los Angeles Times*. Retrieved from http://articles.latimes.com/1987-10-04/local/me-32865_1_cigarette-ad

6. Stuckler, D., & Nestle, M. (2012). Big food, food systems, and global health. *PLoS Medicine, 9*(6), e1001242. Retrieved from doi:10.1371/journal.pmed.1001242

7. Rosenwald, M. (2006, January 22). Why America has to be fat. *Washington Post*. Retrieved from http://www.washingtonpost.com/wp-dyn/content/article/2006/01/21/AR2006012100180.html

8. Isaacs, S., & Swartz, A. (2006). *Banning junk food and soda sales in the state's public schools: A public policy case study*. Los Angeles: California Endowment. Retrieved from http://publichealthadvocacy.org/_PDFs/legislation/banning_junk_food_soda_sales.pdf

9. Carson, R. (1962). *Silent spring*. Boston: Houghton Mifflin.

10. Leonard, A. (2011). *The story of stuff*. New York: Free Press.

11. Delvin, D. (2016, May). Consumers lose $8 billion in fees each year with payday and car-title loans. Retrieved from http://www.responsiblelending.org/media/consumers-lose-8-billion-fees-each-year-payday-and-car-title-loans

12. Donovan, M. (2007, September). D.C. Press conference on payday industry statement. Retrieved from https://www.cohhio.org/files/pdf/nr_09112007.pdf

13. Lazonick, W., & O'Sullivan, M. (2000). Maximizing shareholder value: A new ideology for corporate governance. *Economy and Society, 29*(1), 13–35. doi:10.1080/030851400360541

14. Cohen, L. (n.d.). Lunch with the governor (and the Coke salesman). Retrieved from http://www.preventioninstitute.org/about-us/lp/274-lunch-with-the-governor-and-the-coke-salesman.html

15. Szczypka, G., Wakefield, M.A., Emery, S., Terry-McElrath, Y. M., Flay, B. R., & Chaloupka, F. J. (2007). Working to make an image: An analysis of three Philip Morris corporate image media campaigns. *Tobacco Control, 16*(5), 344–350. Retrieved from doi:10.1136/tc.2007.020412

16. Harris, D. (2001, February 8). Corporate goodwill or tainted money? ABC News. Retrieved from http://abcnews.go.com/WNT/story?id=131249&page=1

17. King, M. L. (1968, April 3). I've been to the moutaintop [Speech Transcript]. Retrieved from http://www.americanrhetoric.com/speeches/mlkivebeentothemountaintop.htm

18. Cortese, A. (2014, August 13). Government grants may help ease business challenges. *The New York Times*. Retrieved from http://www.nytimes.com/2014/08/14/business/smallbusiness/government-grants-may-help-ease-business-challenges.html?_r=0

19. Hancock, T. (2013, July 23). Advocacy is not always popular [Web Log]. Retrieved from https://povertybadforhealth.wordpress.com/2013/07/24/on-government-enemies-list/

20. Baby Milk Action. (n.d.). Nestlé-free zone. Retrieved from http://www.baby-milkaction.org/nestlefree

21. Cohen, L., Chavez, V., & Chehimi, S. (2010). *Prevention is primary: Strategies for community well-being* (2nd ed.). San Francisco: Jossey-Bass.

22. Baby Milk Action. (n.d.). Our mission. Retrieved from http://www.baby-milkaction.org/about-us

23. *The Lancet*. (2016, January 29). Breastfeeding: Achieving the new normal. Retrieved from http://www.thelancet.com/series/breastfeeding.

24. McFadden, A., Masonemail, F., Baker, J., Begin, F., Dykes, F., Grummer-Strawn, L., ... Renfrew, M. J. (2016). Spotlight on infant formula: Coordinated global action needed. *The Lancet, 387*, 413–415. Retrieved from http://www.thelancet.com/journals/lancet/article/PIIS0140-6736(16)00103-3/fulltext

25. Cohen, L., Chavez, V., & Chehimi, S. (2010). *Prevention is primary: Strategies for community well-being*. San Francisco: Jossey-Bass.

26. Personal interview with P. Rundall (2016).

27. Food Chain Workers Alliance. (2014). Walmart at the crossroads: The environmental and labor impact of its food supply chain. Retrieved from http://foodchainworkers.org/wp-content/uploads/2015/06/Walmart-at-the-Crossroads-FINAL-06.04.15.pdf

28. Associate Discount Cards. (n.d.). Walmart. Retrieved from https://www.walmart.com/cservice/discountrules.gsp

29. San Francisco, California, Pro. Ordinance 194-08 (2008).

30. Abrams, R. (2014, September 3). CVS stores stop selling all tobacco products. *The New York Times*. Retrieved from http://www.nytimes.com/2014/09/03/business/cvs-stores-stop-selling-all-tobacco-products.html

31. Camden, M. J. (2006). Campbell announces major sodium reduction plans for top-selling soups. Retrieved from http://www.investor.campbellsoupcompany.com/phoenix.zhtml?c=88650&p=irol-newsArticle_Print&ID=820298&highlight=

32. Brown, E. (2011, July 14). Campbell's to add salt back into Select Harvest soups: Good health doesn't sell. *Los Angeles Times.* Retrieved from http://articles.latimes.com/2011/jul/14/news/la-heb-campbell-soup-sodium-health-20110714

33. Sugary drink facts. (2013). Retrieved from http://www.sugarydrinkfacts.org/resources/SugaryDrinkFACTS_Report_Results.pdf

34. López-Gómez, A., Ros-Chumillas, M., & Belisario-Sánchez, Y. Y. (2010). Packaging and the shelf life of orange juice. In G. R. Robinson (Ed.), *Food packaging and shelf life: A practical guide* (pp. 179–198). Boca Raton, FL: CRC Press.

35. Goetzel, R. Z., Fabius, R., Fabius, D., Roemer, E. C., Thornton, N., Kelly, R. K., & Pelletier, K. R. (2016). The stock performance of C. Everett Koop Award winners compared with the Standard & Poor's 500 Index. *Journal of Occupational and Environmental Medicine, 58*(1), 9–15. Retrieved from http://journals.lww.com/joem/Fulltext/2016/01000/The_Stock_Performance_of_C__Everett_Koop_Award.3.aspx

Chapter 10

1. Newport, F. (2010, December 2). Most Americans take doctor's advice without second opinion. Retrieved from http://www.gallup.com/poll/145025/americans-doctor-advice-without-second-opinion.aspx

2. Pearson, S. D., & Raeke, L. H. (2000). Patients' trust in physicians: Many theories, few measures, and little data. *Journal of General Internal Medicine, 15*(7), 509–513. http://doi.org/10.1046/j.1525-1497.2000.11002.x

3. Kantrajian, H. (2014, May 30). An unhealthy system. Retrieved from http://www.usnews.com/opinion/articles/2014/05/30/no-the-us-doesnt-have-the-best-health-care-system-in-the-world

4. Tandon, A., Murray, C. J. L., Lauer, J. A., & Evans, D. B. (n.d.). Measuring overall health system performance for 191 countries. GPE Discussion Paper Series no. 30. Retrieved from http://www.who.int/healthinfo/paper30.pdf

5. Murray, C. J. L., Lauer, J., Tandon, A., & Frenk, J. (n.d.). Overall health system achievement for 191 countries. Discussion Paper Series No. 28. Retrieved from http://www.who.int/healthinfo/paper28.pdf

6. World Health Organization. (2000). *Health systems: Improving performance.* World Health Report 2000. Geneva: Author. Retrieved from http://www.who.int/whr/2000/en/whr00_en.pdf

7. Newport, Most Americans take doctor's advice.

8. World Health Organization. (n.d.). Health Impact Assessment: The determinants of health. Retrieved from http://www.who.int/hia/evidence/doh/en/

9. Prevention Institute. (2003, November). Making the case with THRIVE: Background research on community determinants of health. Retrieved from http://www.preventioninstitute.org/component/jlibrary/article/id-96/127.html

10. Scitovsky, A. A. (2005). The high cost of dying: What do the data show? *The Milbank Quarterly, 83*(4), 825–841. Retrieved from http://doi.org/10.1111/j.1468-0009.2005.00402.x

11. Schoen, C., Doty, M. M., Collins, S. R., & Holmgren, A. L. (2005). Insured but not protected: How many adults are underinsured? *Health Affairs, 24*(4), 1187.

12. Otto, M. (2014, April 8). Lack of access to dental care leads to expensive emergency room care. Retrieved from http://healthjournalism.org/blog/2014/04/lack-of-access-to-dental-care-leads-to-expensive-emergency-room-care/

13. Harmon K. (2010, April 16). Health insurers make big bucks from Big Macs. Retrieved from http://blogs.scientificamerican.com/observations/health-insurers-make-big-bucks-from-big-macs/

14. Kiersh, A. (2009, July 6). Health care stakeholders send ex-lawmakers, staffers to Capitol Hill. Retrieved from http://www.opensecrets.org/news/2009/07/health-care-stakeholders-send/

15. Pickert K. (2010, February 4). The unsustainable U.S. health care system. Retrieved from http://swampland.time.com/2010/02/04/the-unsustainable-u-s-health-care-system/

16. Martin, A. B., Lassman, D., Washington, B., Catlin, A., & National Health Expenditure Accounts Team. (2012, January). Growth in US health spending remained slow in 2010; health share of gross domestic product was unchanged from 2009. *Health Affairs, 31*(1), 208–219.

17. The World Bank. (n.d.). Health expenditure, total (% of GDP). Retrieved from http://data.worldbank.org/indicator/SH.XPD.TOTL.ZS

18. County of Los Angeles, Department of Parks and Recreation. (2012, October 12). Parks after dark. Paper presented at the Health Education Practice Conference, Los Angeles. Retrieved from http://publichealth.lacounty.gov/hea/HEPracticeConference/2012/Fischer_ParksAfterDarkFinal.pdf

19. Maciosek, M., Coffield, A. B., Flottemesch, T. J., Edwards, N. M. & Solberg, L. I. (2010). Greater use of preventive services in U.S. health care could save lives at little or no cost. *Health Affairs, 29*(9), 1656–1660. Retrieved from doi:10.1377/hlthaff.2008.0701

20. Laff, M. (2015, May 13). Family physician salaries up but still trail those of subspecialists. Retrieved from http://www.aafp.org/news/practice-professional-issues/20150513salaryreport.html

21. Durso, L. E., & Gates, G. J. (2012). *Serving our youth: Findings from a national survey of service providers working with lesbian, gay, bisexual, and transgender youth*

who are homeless or at risk of becoming homeless. Los Angeles: Williams Institute with True Colors Fund and Palette Fund. Retrieved from http://williamsinstitute.law.ucla.edu/wp-content/uploads/Durso-Gates-LGBT-Homeless-Youth-Survey-July-2012.pdf

22. Kosciw, J. G., Greytak, E. A., Bartkiewicz, M. J., Boesen, M. J., & Palmer, N. A. (2012). *The 2011 National School Climate Survey: The experiences of lesbian, gay, bisexual and transgender youth in our nation's schools.* New York: GLSEN.

23. Ibid.

24. DHCS: Research and Analytic Studies Division. (2015). Understanding Medi-Cal's high cost populations (PowerPoint).

25. Prevention Institute. (2011, May). Fact sheets: Links between violence and chronic diseases. Retrieved from http://www.preventioninstitute.org/component/jlibrary/article/id-301/127.html

26. Kohn, L. T., Corrigan, J. M., & Donaldson, M. S. (Eds.). (2000). *To err is human: Building a safer health system,* Vol. 6. Washington, DC: National Academies Press. Retrieved from http://iom.nationalacademies.org/Reports/1999/To-Err-is-Human-Building-A-Safer-Health-System.aspx

27. James, J. T. (2013). A new, evidence-based estimate of patient harms associated with hospital care. *Journal of Patient Safety, 9*(3), 122–128. Retrieved from http://journals.lww.com/journalpatientsafety/Fulltext/2013/09000/A_New,_Evidence_based_Estimate_of_Patient_Harms.2.aspx

28. Centers for Disease Control and Prevention. (n.d.). Mortality multiple cause micro-data files. Retrieved from http://www.cdc.gov/nchs/data/nvsr/nvsr64/nvsr64_02.pdf

29. Magill, S. S., Edwards, J. R., Bamberg, W., Beldavs, Z. G., Dumyati, G., Kainer, M. A., ... Ray, S. M. (2014). Multistate point-prevalence survey of health care-associated infections. *New England Journal of Medicine, 370*(13), 1198–1208. Retrieved from http://www.nejm.org/doi/full/10.1056/NEJMoa1306801

30. Johnson, J. A., & Bootman, J. L. (1995). Drug related morbidity and mortality: A cost-of-illness model. *Archives of Internal Medicine, 155*(18), 1949–1956.

31. Shepherd G., Mohorn, P., Yacoub, K., & May D. W. (2012). Adverse drug reaction deaths reported in United States vital statistics, 1999–2006. Retrieved from http://www.ncbi.nlm.nih.gov/pubmed/22253191

32. US General Accounting Office. (2002). *Prescription drugs: FDA oversight of direct to consumer advertising has limitations.* Washington, DC: Author.

33. Ross B. (2009, June 19). More macaroni, bon voyage Viagra: Why prescription medicines should not be advertised. *The Huffington Post.* Retrieved from http://www.huffingtonpost.com/brian ross/more macaroni bon voyage_b_205304.html

34. Substance Abuse and Mental Health Service Administration. (n.d.). Highlights of the 2011 Drug Abuse Warning Network (DAWN) findings on drug-related emergency department visits. Retrieved from http://www.samhsa.gov/data/2k13/DAWN127/sr127-DAWN-highlights.htm

35. Centers for Disease Control and Prevention. (n.d.). Mortality data. Retrieved from http://www.cdc.gov/nchs/deaths.htm

36. Breu, G. (1981, September 14). Dr. Bob Sanders prescribes car seats to save kids in crashes. Retrieved from http://www.people.com/people/archive/article/0,,20080205,00.html

37. Associated Press. (1984, October 10). 14 San Francisco sex clubs told to close to curb AIDS. Retrieved from http://www.nytimes.com/1984/10/10/us/14-san-francisco-sex-clubs-told-to-close-to-curb-aids.html

38. Prothrow-Stith, D., & Weissman, M. (1991). *Deadly consequences.* New York: HarperCollins.

39. Mikkelsen, L., Cohen, L., & Frankowski, S. (2014). Engaging health care in building healthy communities. *National Civic Review, 103*(1), 57–59. Retrieved from http://dx.doi.org/10.1002/ncr.21179

40. Cantor, J., Cohen, L., Mikkelsen, L., Pañares, R., Srikantharajah, J., & Valdovinos, E. (2011). *Community-centered health homes: Bridging the gap between health services and community prevention.* Oakland, CA: Prevention Institute.

41. Waters, R. (2013, December 12). In South Los Angeles, a bold plan to address health disparities. Retrieved from http://www.forbes.com/sites/robwaters/2013/12/12/in-south-los-angeles-a-bold-plan-to-address-health-disparities/#2715e4857a0b6d29fdba59d5

42. Waters, R. (2013, November 26). *It's all in the data: Cincinnati Children's Hospital gets wonky to transform the health of its community.* Retrieved from http://www.forbes.com/sites/robwaters/2013/11/26/its-all-in-the-data-cincinnati-childrens-hospital-gets-wonky-to-transform-a-communitys-health/2/#2715e4857a0b780f93da771f

43. Jack Geiger, M.D., M.Sc., ScD. (2014, March 10). Retrieved from http://wearepublichealthproject.org/interview/jack-geiger/

44. Lightwood, J., & Glantz, S. A. (2013). The effect of the California Tobacco Control Program on smoking prevalence, cigarette consumption, and health-care costs: 1989–2008. *PLoS ONE, 8*(2), e47145.

45. Gottlieb, L. (2010, August 23). Funding healthy society helps cure health care. *SFGate.* Retrieved from http://www.sfgate.com/opinion/openforum/article/Funding-healthy-society-helps-cure-health-care-3177542.php

46. Finkelstein M. (2015, October 20). Tiearona low dog elevates the meaning of "integrative medicine." *The Huffington Post.* Retrieved from http://www.huffingtonpost.com/michael-finkelstein-md/tiearona-low-dog-elevates_b_8334708.html

47. White, R. (2015, March 4). Why "health doesn't equal health care." Retrieved from http://www.centerforhealthjournalism.org/2015/03/03/why-health-doesnt-equal-health-care

Chapter 11

1. Executive Office of the President of the United States. (2013). Impacts and costs of the October 2013 federal government shutdown. Retrieved from https://www.whitehouse.gov/sites/default/files/omb/reports/impacts-and-costs-of-october-2013-federal-government-shutdown-report.pdf

2. US Census Bureau. (n.d.). Quick facts Flint City, Michigan. Retrieved from http://www.census.gov/quickfacts/table/LFE041214/2629000,00

3. US Department of Health and Human Services. (n.d.). Laws and policies. Retrieved from http://betobaccofree.hhs.gov/laws/

4. US Food and Drug Administration. (2015). Toxic Substances Control Act (TSCA) and federal facilities. Retrieved from http://www.epa.gov/enforcement/toxic-substances-control-act-tsca-and-federal-facilities

5. O'Neil, B. (2002, January/February). Accidents or crashes: Highway safety and William Haddon Jr. *Contingencies*, 30–32.

6. Jones, B., Dellinger, A., & Wallace, D. (1999). Achievements in public health, 1900–1999. Motor vehicle safety: A 20th century public health achievement. *Morbidity and Mortality Weekly Report, 48*, 369–374.

7. Swerdloff, A. (2015, June 30). How Coney Island became the unlikely birthplace of outdoor dining. Retrieved from https://munchies.vice.com/en/articles/how-coney-island-became-the-unlikely-birthplace-of-outdoor-dining

8. Blackmar, E., & Rosenzweig, R. (n.d.). History. Retrieved from http://www.centralpark.com/guide/history.html

9. Beveridge, C. (n.d.). Frederick Law Olmsted Sr.: Landscape architect, author, conservationist (1822–1903). Retrieved from http://www.olmsted.org/the-olmsted-legacy/frederick-law-olmsted-sr

10. Maggs, L. (2003). Newsmaker: Baby versus the giant—Patti Rundall, policy director, Baby Milk Action. *Third Sector*. Retrieved from http://www.thirdsector.co.uk/Channels/Fundraising/Article/619829/NEWSMAKER-Baby-versus-giant--Patti-Rundall-Policy-director-Baby-Milk-Action

11. Rich, A. (1977). Natural resources. Retrieved from http://poetsorg.tumblr.com/post/20464216572/adrienne-rich-natural-resources-1977-my

12. Cure Violence. (2014). *Annual Report 2014*. Retrieved from http://cureviolence.org/wp-content/uploads/2015/06/Cure-Violence-Annual-Report-2014.pdf

13. NFL. (2015, August 12). The NFL's response to domestic violence and sexual assault. Retrieved from http://www.nfl.com/news/story/0ap3000000439286/article/the-nfls-response-to-domestic-violence-and-sexual-assault

14. Healey, M. (2015, December 7). AG Healey Announces 98 High Schools Across the State to Participate in Game Change: The Patriots Anti-Violence Partnership. Retrieved from http://www.mass.gov/ago/news-and-updates/press-releases/2015/2015-12-07-game-change-schools.html

15. Genesee Valley Health Partnership. "second step violence prevention." Retrieved from http://www.gvhp.org/second-step-violence-prevention.html
16. Gerstein, A. (2014). *Executive director's message.* Retrieved from http://gardnercenter.stanford.edu/about_jgc/welcome.html
17. Heart, A. (n.d.). Quotes by Amelia Earhart. Retrieved from http://www.ameliaearhart.com/about/quotes.html
18. Benowitz, N. L., Blum, A., Braithwaite, R. L., & Castro, F. G. (2014). *Tobacco use among US racial/ethnic minority groups: African Americans, American Indians and Alaska natives, Asian Americans and Pacific islanders, and Hispanics: A report of the Surgeon General.* Atlanta: Centers for Disease Control and Prevention.
19. Healton, C., & Nelson, K. (2004). Reversal of misfortune: Viewing tobacco as a social justice issue. *American Journal of Public Health, 94*(2), 186–191.
20. Feinberg, S. (2012, December 2). Cigarette price increases don't burden low-income New Yorkers, smoking does. *The Huffington Post.* Retrieved from http://www.huffingtonpost.com/sheelah-a-feinberg/cigarette-price-increases_b_1934038.html

WEB COMPANION AND DISCUSSION QUESTIONS

www.preventiondiaries.org

For more in-depth background and up-to date information and resources, visit *Prevention Diaries'* comprehensive web companion at www.preventiondiaries.org.

- Find discussion questions to use in your classroom or for your book club.
- Explore expanded references and resources.
- Watch videos and listen to podcasts.
- Learn about recent developments and upcoming opportunities to support prevention and equity.

INDEX